REALITY FITNESS

Website addresses provided in this book were accurate at the time it went to press.

Cover Design: Nathan Smith
Editor: Erinne Sevigny Adachi
Fitness Photography: Claudine Lavoie

First Printing, 2017
ISBN: 978-0-9952351-0-6

Acacia Fitness
Edmonton, Alberta, Canada
www.acaciafitness.com
www.realityfitnessbook.com

DISCLAIMER

The information provided reflects the author's experience and opinions and is designed to help you make informed decisions about your body and health. The suggestions for specific foods and exercises in this program are not intended to replace appropriate or necessary medical care.

Before starting any exercise regimen, always consult your physician. Ask for a physical stress test. If any recommendations in this book contradict your physician's advice, be sure to consult him or her before proceeding. The mention of specific products, organizations, companies, or authorities in this book does not imply endorsement by the author, nor does the mention of specific organizations, companies, or authorities imply that they endorse this book. The author disclaims any liability or loss, personal or otherwise, that is incurred as a result, directly or indirectly, of the use and applications of any of the contents of this publication.

REALITY FITNESS

ANGELA DEJONG

For my Favourite Dad

TABLE OF CONTENTS

AUTHOR'S NOTE

My name is Angela deJong, and I am a certified personal trainer and bona-fide fitness and health enthusiast. My passions in life are travel and fitness, so I combine the two no matter where in the world I find myself. Whether I am working out with a trainer to the stars in a private New York City apartment, having a pushup contest inside a mud hut deep in the Anti-Atlas mountains of Morocco, desperately trying to keep up to an Ethiopian soccer team on a morning run, doing pushups in a Cameroon hostel while trying to keep cockroaches from crawling on my bare hands, or taking the final steps to another summit—I've climbed, hiked, or trained everywhere I have visited. Fitness and health have provided me with the confidence and ability to see and do some of the most extraordinary things on the planet. It's how I meet local people, learn new fitness techniques, and simply better myself as a person and fitness trainer.

It has not always been easy, though. Maintaining a fitness and healthy eating routine requires planning and perseverance, but it's worth it! The results of all that planning and perseverance keep me healthy so that I can actually do all the activities I want to do. My lifestyle provides me the energy and strength to live the life I want.

Your story might be similar, or maybe you're looking to live a fuller life closer to home—to be fit enough to keep up with your kids and grandkids, to improve your golf game, or simply to wake up each day with more vitality.

I wrote Reality Fitness to celebrate the individual achievements of my clients, my friends, my family, and in particular my dad. All have successfully changed their lives one step at a time using this proven method of sustained weight management. Clear insight into the reality of what it takes to actually lose weight and get healthy was my goal in developing this program. Losing weight is not a linear process—there will be ups and downs along the way. But with a consistently executed plan, your goal is attainable. I wanted to share this method with others who may be in a place of frustration or confusion about how to get back to health or to lose the extra weight and keep it off, while not giving up part of the things that make life worth living. Abstaining from the moments in our lives and culture that are celebrated with food, be that cake for your birthday or champagne at a retirement party, is not necessary to achieve results. You do not need to be perfect. Rather, daily habitual change, food boundaries, and a positive mindset are key. Weight loss, health, and fitness do not have to be "all or nothing." You can still lose weight and eat cake!

I understand the investment of money—and more importantly time—when you purchase a book and implement a new fitness and nutrition routine. Thank you for choosing Reality Fitness among all the books out there. I am so excited for your weight loss journey to begin. There will be triumphs and struggles, and that is okay. Just like climbing mountains, this process is one step at a time. Have patience, be deliberate in your steps, and pay attention to your surroundings. Revel in the journey and the summit is inevitable.

PROGRAM GENESIS

HOW A FITNESS TRAINER AND NUTRITION NUT HELPED HER DAD DROP THE WEIGHT, FOR GOOD!

My dad, Terry Thachuk, was the proverbial poster man of the typical North American trying to lose weight. He was smart and aware of the many things he should do. He was especially motivated to try several different methods that promise a quick slim down. Constantly thinking about his number on the scale, he was always watching, reading, or listening for the latest fitness and nutrition hype, and absorbing it all in an attempt to create the "ultimate weight loss program" . . . that he would start on Monday. He was accomplished in so many areas of his life, but his weight was the one area he could not seem to get under control. It was frustrating, almost depressing at times.

My dad was no stranger to hard work. Growing up in a rural Albertan community as the youngest of seven brothers, he started working at the age of twelve at his dad's army surplus auto sales business. By seventeen he was living away from his parents with one of his brothers in a small apartment in the city. There was not much of an opportunity to be a teenager. With bills and school and work, my dad was ahead of his years when it came to responsibilities. It was around this time, he tells me, that he picked up his first pack of cigarettes.

My dad continued to succeed in his work over the years, and with that came more pressure. This led to an increase in smoking and a lot of coffee consumed to "manage stress and provide some energy." My mom would pack wonderful lunches for him and they often came back at the end of the day untouched because "there was no time to eat." As any shift worker could tell you, it was a challenge to get into any kind of routine. It was not uncommon to see Dad "rest his eyes" after supper or to see him attempt to stay up a full 24 hours in order to reset his biological clock before his next shift. My dad adapted to surviving on very little sleep, to living off coffee and cigarettes and usually a single huge meal for the day.

This lifestyle was breaking pretty much every health rule we know today, but back then, my dad was young and super thin, and it appeared as if it had no effect on him. In fact, he wore it as a badge of honour.

> "I can eat whatever I want, however much I want, and I never gain weight," he would say. (Sound familiar?)

As the awareness of smoking-related health risks became prevalent, it became more difficult for my dad to smoke in certain locations. Restaurants, the mall, and even work were all eventually restricted. But that didn't stop him from his three packages of cigarettes per day (that's seventy five smokes, by the way).

Eventually (and not surprisingly) my dad had a few heart scares, one resulting in an emergency visit, several months of debilitating vertigo, and circulation problems for years. These were not enough to convince him to quit. Instead, it was a short video he saw of himself giving a presentation where his speech was interrupted every two minutes in an effort to release the phlegm from his throat. He was mortified by how he sounded and looked. That was the moment my dad decided to quit smoking.

He conquered his addiction using the patch, initially, and then through sheer determination. As many former smokers do, my dad turned to a new habit to replace his old one. Instead of turning to eating, though, my dad turned to juicing after seeing an infomercial that inspired him to get healthy. He was excited about the opportunity to "get all the years of tar and build-up out of his system" by offsetting this with powerful antioxidants in fresh juice he would prepare himself. He would make up for years of abuse to his body with as many fresh fruits as he could. How many glasses of juice does it take to replace 75 cigarettes a day? Let's just say a few too many!

After nearly six months of no smoking and copious glasses of freshly squeezed fruit, my dad was so excited to visit the doctor and tell him about his perceived positive lifestyle changes. While he knew he had put on some extra pounds ("That's only natural after you stop smoking," he'd say), he was shocked to find out it was 39 of them. And not only that, he was told for the first time that he had high blood pressure . . . so high his physician suggested medication until he could lose some of the weight. This left him frustrated and confused. "Fruit is healthy and low in calories, so why have I gained weight?"

This was the start of his weight loss journey, as my dad tried as many fad diets and quick fixes as he could to lose the weight as quickly as possible. He was in a constant cycle of trying something new for a few days or weeks and then giving up and moving to the next plan, never really committing to a program for long enough to reap the benefits, desperate to get the weight off, and perhaps with a lack of belief in either the program or even himself. But maybe it's best if I let him tell the story from his point of view.

Take it away, Dad.

T-MAN'S STRAIGHT TALK

Yo, yo, yo! My name is Terry. I'm Ang's rock-star dad, and I guess this is my story of how I went from fat ass to fit. You'll see me pop in during your phases with some straight talk and some of my best tips to help you make it through each challenge in one piece. I'll warn you right now: This was not a cake walk, but if you want it to, it will work. It gets easier over time, but the entire process will challenge you week after week, slowly edging you out of your comfort zone until that new zone becomes what's comfortable! I was unsure of what to expect, but after the program was complete I felt proud of what I accomplished. I finally committed to one plan and it worked. I no longer felt the guilt of eating something "bad" or eating too much or continually feeling like a failure because I set the bar for change too high. I felt healthy and excited to get out and try new activities. I knew that I needed to lose the weight for health reasons, but I never imagined how it would impact my state of mind, outlook on life, and overall happiness. The effort you put in is absolutely worth it!

Ang already filled you in on the back story. Let me pick it back up from the first time I decided to make some moves toward a healthier and lighter me—that's after the whole juice debacle. Ang is cringing right now reading this fearing that I am making it sound like juice and fruit are bad for you. Let's be clear: they are not, and they won't make you fat, if you eat them in reasonable quantities. But she was right to caution me yet again when on Skype I held up two giant bags of fruit from the store and told her it all was my juice for the day.

It was January, a few years back. I can't remember when exactly, but I was on a rampage! Diane, my wife, and I cleaned the house out of all snacks, bought fresh foods and new bikes (we live in a climate where biking in January is possible). That was it. I'd had enough. I was going to lose weight and get off the high blood pressure medication my doctor prescribed. The game plan was that every day Diane and I would ride our neighbourhood loop (about 10 miles) and eat as little food as possible. And definitely no juice since learning that it was the "healthy" juice that caused all the problems in the first place. I figured my energy intake (food) would be less than my energy output (exercise), so my weight loss formula would be the cat's ass. I did this with Diane for about three days despite feeling kind of dizzy on the bike and veering randomly across the road onto the curb from time to time. And let's not even get into what a sensational mood I was in during those days. In my mind it was worth the agony to drop the weight in a few weeks time. But after those three days, I stepped on the scale and saw no change! I was astonished and felt utterly defeated. It didn't make any sense. I had not eaten anything bad in three days and I was exercising. How was I not losing weight?

Lucky for me, my favourite daughter (my only daughter) is a personal trainer and could probably answer my questions. I called her asking for a few ideas on what I could do to move this along. She suggested I start with one small step and then add on incrementally once I felt comfortable. But that wouldn't do it for me. I had more urgency than she did, so I pushed for a few more ideas on what to do. Every time I called her like this, she obliged her old man. I'd get off the phone feeling motivated to start implementing her latest tips—and I would for a couple of days—and then I would stop. Again. And Again. This went on for a few months. I refused to hear what she was trying to tell me: *Slow. Down.*

Daily, I would come up with new reasons as to why I wasn't finding success, and lo and behold, I'd find a new solution on a TV program or in a magazine or on the radio. I'd always call Ang for her opinion, and she was never negative about the ideas, but she kept suggesting I slow things down and focus on one change at a time. Slow things down? Why on earth would I do that? I had a gut to lose ASAP! It made no sense to me to slow things down. Quite the opposite. I needed to ramp things up! So I increased our bike ride from 10 miles to 12 miles a day (because more is always better), and I made a commitment to never have juice again, and I read somewhere that almonds are good for you so I had 10 of those everyday, and I also heard that chicken was good for you so I started eating that almost every supper, and I bought an ab crunch machine to target my love handles with the intention of using it twice as often as the directions recommended for miracle speed results. My new plan was boring, and gave me a back ache like you wouldn't believe, but I was certain it would be effective if I could just keep going. That week I lost a pound. I was torturing myself and that was all I got?! One. Lousy. Pound.

Ticked off, I rang up my favourite daughter again and asked her to put together a detailed meal plan for me. I was certain if I could just follow a meal plan to the letter, the weight would fall off. Ang said that although it looked simple to follow with the foods I needed listed, in the correct quantities, it was not realistic to do it for the rest of my life. I figured I could just do it long enough to get the weight off and then I could eat other stuff later on. Now, I am a pretty disciplined guy, but yet again I was only able to follow the eating plan for a little over a week. One dinner out with friends, and I had no idea what to order off the menu because my meal plan options were not on there.

The frustration of not having perfect execution would inevitably derail me. Why couldn't I stick with my plan?

Today I realize it was because I lacked the understanding of why I was eating those kinds of foods and how they each affected my health, energy, and metabolism. It was easy to make my own "adjustments" to the plan when I didn't understand the importance of the details put into it.

The next time Ang answered her phone it was to a frantic and infuriated father. I was sick of chicken, her mother wanted to throw her bike off a cliff, and I had come across a new app that told me that almonds were high in calories, so I didn't want to eat them anymore. Ang went to reply, but I wasn't done venting. I started reading off my list: I wanted a few new tips for my exercise, and one or two quick fat loss snack ideas. Had she heard about that "revolutionary" supplement for belly fat, and should I buy it? Also! Diane was reading a book that had some crazy exercise on a strappy thing with a ball, and it was supposed to be the greatest stomach workout ever. Should I get one? And also: how do those fat people on that fat show lose so much weight in one week? And why with all my efforts was my belly getting bigger—it was going to start affecting my golf game. I was serious now about taking action, so maybe she could give me an ab workout that I could do everyday that wouldn't kill my back like that horrendous contraption? And last on the list, exactly how many beers on Fridays are too many?

Sadly, it was years before I finally admitted that none of my approaches were working. I'm sure some of you can relate. To move forward, I would have to let go of all the quick-fix promises, the confusing and conflicting tidbits of information I had accumulated over the years with regards to fitness, health, and weight loss. I decided on a detox—but not that kind of detox. Heck, I'd tried those already and look where it got me! I put away my fitness magazines, stopped watching all the infomercials, and stopped visiting supplement stores. And—again—I called Ang. I was ready to slow down.

"What is my first and only step to take right now?" I asked.

Going forward with Ang's approach, I would focus on one nutrition and exercise challenge every two weeks. If I could manage being 80% compliant, then Ang would advance me to the next step. I was still nervous that it was not going to work or that it would take forever to lose the weight, but obviously my way of doing things wasn't working either. It had been years, after all. When the process finally started I felt relieved to have structure, simplicity, and a tangible target every day. I had a plan and it was either do X or do not do X . . . simple as that. *And* it was a plan that still allowed me to have a beer without feeling guilty about it!

I repeat: BEER IS ALLOWED IN THIS PROGRAM.

With every new challenge, I was able to measure my compliance on the tracking sheets Ang gave me to keep me accountable. Before, my success had always been based on how much weight I had lost. Now, my success was based on the execution of the necessary steps to earn the weight loss. I just had to trust the process and do it.

And don't worry. Ang didn't spend all these years writing a book to tell you I failed! You'll get to see how I did every step of the way throughout the book. There's a happy ending to this story, and you'll have one too, if you do the work. Ultimately, I gained the healthiest body I have ever known through good nutrition, learning how to exercise, and discovering that there is something deeply rewarding to all this being healthy shit that goes beyond losing body fat and gaining muscle.

In the end, my weight loss was a bi-product of the success in all the small steps that brought me to my current level of health and fitness.

When I write my whole story out, I see now how desperate I was and so confused all at the same time. No wonder I was not finding success . . . I lacked focus. I was trying to change everything all at once! And I sure as hell wasn't being patient about waiting for the results. Sometimes I wish I had just listened to Ang right from the beginning and saved myself all that stress and frustration. But on the flip side, it was all that frustration that eventually led me to appreciate what it truly takes to make a successful, long-lasting change.

TERRY'S TIPS

1. Be patient. It is likely to take several weeks of work before you'll start to see results. That doesn't mean the program isn't working or that you're doing something wrong. Keep going!

2. Don't skip ahead. The challenges are in a particular order and move slow on purpose so that each becomes a foundational aspect to your

lifestyle. Don't risk it all toppling over because you tried to add a new habit on top of one that wasn't cemented yet.

3. Don't skip reading the mindset section. That might be the most important factor to your success.

4. Have fun. This book is full of opportunities to make things interesting, whether it's making yourself some playlists for your workouts or trying new foods and recipes.

5. Start saving some extra cash. By the time this is done, you're gonna need some new pants.

My dad was the inspiration for *Reality Fitness*. He proved that small, incremental steps add up over time, and that perfection is not necessary for success. Now he's retired and living it up! Instead of frantic phone calls with questions about how he can quickly drop pounds, I get text messages from him about how many times he's climbed the stairs at his hotel or how much money he won on the golf course.

My dad, beer in hand, is now the poster man for a fitness program that works. Other clients who have gone through the program have married, started families, moved to new locations, run marathons, climbed mountains, changed careers, started businesses, travelled, and started dreaming again.

This is what life is about . . . think about *living* instead of about when you are going to lose the weight or obsessing over what you can and cannot eat or how fat you look in your pants.

> When you feel proud of who you are and what you have accomplished, you make decisions for your life rather than having life and circumstance decide for you.

Through this book, it is my ambition to empower you to see your potential so that you are self-motivated to take the incremental steps necessary to live a healthier, fuller life. Let's get started!

YOUR MINDSET: YOUR KEY TO SUCCESS

If there is one thing that separates the successful from the unsuccessful, it is mindset. Without question, a positive mindset is the "magic pill" to weight loss. But having a positive mindset isn't as easy as flipping a switch. Following are critical components to developing a positive mindset for success in the *Reality Fitness* weight loss program.

1. MAKE A DECISION INSTEAD OF A GOAL

I find the word goal is overused, and it is not necessarily the best term for this program. In my opinion, the word provides you with an out if you find the target you are working toward is too hard, or you get tired, or you have another excuse not to continue. I like the word decision. By using the word decision, you are telling yourself and everyone around you that you have drawn the line in the sand. This is what you are doing—no questions asked—no matter what it takes. You still have a target you are working toward, but you are using a more definitive word about your intentions to get there.

Compare the two following examples and consider how you react to them.

"I'm setting a goal to lose thirty pounds."

Vs.

"I have decided to lose thirty pounds."

Both of these sound very positive, but the second one suggests that this person means business. The second line feels more actionable.

> Words have power. I challenge you to pay attention to the words you use when you talk about what you are going to do to get healthy and fit.

Words such as *hope, wish, maybe, tomorrow,* don't put you in a mindset ready for change. Words such as *decision, will, am, now, choice*—these set you up for success.

Putting your foot down and proclaiming a decision can be intimidating at first, but it holds you more accountable. Once you make your decision, you will feel empowered and motivated to do what is necessary to reach your target. The following are some important factors that will make a difference in choosing and sticking to your decisions.

CLARITY IS KEY

Your decision should be clear in terms of what you are going to do (or want) and how you are going to do it. For example: "I am going to lose thirty pounds and I've decided to use this book to get me there." Write your decision down!

> If your decision lacks clarity, you will lack focus and motivation, especially during the more challenging times.

It is okay if your final decision feels daunting. Focusing on small decisions along the way will reduce that overwhelming feeling, and those small decisions are laid out for you one by one in this book to help eliminate the complexity of losing weight.

KNOW THE ALTERNATIVE

For every decision there is the alternative. When you write down your decision, incorporate the alternative to reinforce why you are doing this. For example: "I have decided to lose thirty pounds instead of feeling bad about myself everyday and putting myself at risk for serious health issues."

TRACK IT

As mentioned, this system provides you with all the small steps to get you to where you want to be. It even includes the tracking sheets you'll need, but actually using them is up to you.

> Tracking your progress is crucial to keeping yourself motivated.

It allows you to learn about yourself and your habits as you work to change them, and it provides concrete proof of your effort and successes along the way—a huge contributing factor to your momentum through this program!

DON'T SET A TIMELINE

Contrary to a lot of goal setting concepts, for this program a timeline is not required and would in fact be detrimental. Learning any new skill (yes, nutrition habits and exercise are indeed skills) takes time, trial and error, and consistency. Many people try to skip steps or rush the process to try and lose the weight as quickly as possible. Inevitably this pattern leads to a feeling of deprivation or feelings of major discomfort that are not sustainable. The entire reason for this program is to help you lose the weight, but it is more importantly to help you keep the weight off for good. Listen to how you feel throughout the program. Ask yourself from time to time: "Can I continue to maintain these changes for the next five years, ten years, etc.?" If the answer is yes, then you are ready to move on to the next stage of the book. A little discomfort is normal. That hanging-on-by-the-skin-of-your-teeth feeling is pushing yourself too far, too fast. If this happens, take a step back, regroup, then move forward. When it comes to this program, that means taking an extra week (or more) to really nail a new habit instead of pushing on to the next one before really being ready. There is nothing wrong with waiting until you are comfortable before moving forward.

2. PRESENCE

The past is over, and soon today will be the past too. Focusing on the past and all the poor choices you made to put yourself in this position will not help you. By taking action today you are creating a better past, a better present, and an even better future. Use your past as motivation for change and as a learning opportunity to acknowledge that what you were doing has not been working, but do not focus on it too much or you risk feeling poorly about yourself.

Focusing too much on the future can also hinder your success. Yes, it is inspiring to visualize a healthier, fitter version of yourself, but if you omit the focus on the incremental steps that will eventually lead you there, it can feel like that newer version of yourself is an eternity away. This can kill momentum and lead to giving up.

It's time to focus on the here and now.

3. PATIENCE

The catalyst of change isn't often when things are doing all right. Rather, it is almost as if things need to get bad enough that the proverbial straw breaks the camel's back and we decide to overhaul a thousand things at once in the hopes that change for the better happens as fast as possible. I call this the *frantic state*. Sometimes the frantic state is a good place to be in. It at least alarms us enough to embrace the fact that a change needs to happen. However, panic can fuel the frantic state even further causing not only a total lack of focus and disorganization right off the get go, but more stress than is needed. Alternatively, the frantic state can cause paralysis. If you become overwhelmed with the change that you have blown up in your mind as this huge, how-can-this-possibly-be-accomplished task, you will not even know where to begin . . . so you won't.

> Remember: gaining the weight took time, and losing it will also take time.

Focus on the day-by-day and celebrate your achievements—it is critical to staying on track and motivated. Eventually (and faster than it might feel, at first) those days add up to weeks, months, and years of better decisions that lead to a lighter, healthier body.

4. REFRAME NEGATIVE SELF-TALK

Change is challenging and downright difficult at times. If you tell yourself you cannot do something or that you are bad at it, you will believe this and ultimately despise doing it. You're likely to quit before you are ahead. One of the most important pieces to this program is eliminating negative self-talk. Avoid saying: "I'm tired; I'm sick; I don't feel like it; I'm weak; I hate this; I'm fat; I'm lazy; I'm disgusting; I'm a failure; I don't deserve this; I can't . . ." The list goes on and on. If you beat yourself up throughout this process, it is going to be very difficult to continue until the end. And if you do make it to the end, it sure is not going to leave a very positive mark on you to make it a long-lasting part of your life. Who wants to be treated like that? Would you ever say these things to anyone else? What if your best friend or son or daughter said those things to themselves . . . what would you say?

I am not asking you to lie to yourself. I am asking you to change your attitude toward yourself and your efforts. You may not even realize you are doing this, so start paying attention or get others to point it out to you.

When you catch yourself engaging in negative thoughts, reframe it into something positive or motivating.

Here are some examples I have heard from clients:

"These pushups would be so much easier if my stomach wasn't so fat and gross."
Great, that is super motivating, isn't it? OR
"My stomach is fat, but I am doing something about it."

"I did everything I was supposed to and lost no weight this week. What is the point of doing all of this then?"
That's one way to look at it. OR
"I did everything I was supposed to this week and I am one week healthier because of it. The healthier my body becomes, the sooner the weight will start to drop."

5. AVOID COMPARISONS

We all do it from time to time, but when it comes to fitness and health, comparisons are not always helpful motivators. Your weight loss journey is unique. Some people lose weight faster than others. Some people have more barriers to overcome than others. Some people have more free time, less stress, more supportive family and friends. In other words, just because someone you know lost a lot of weight fast does not mean you are a failure if it takes you longer to accomplish a similar benchmark.

It does not matter what kind of workouts other people are doing. Your workouts have been designed with a purpose . . . that purpose is for you to lose weight. It does not matter how hard someone else's workout is; it does not matter what kind of equipment other people are using or what new fitness gadget is out these days. All that matters is that you are fitting in workouts and doing the best that you can when you are there. There is always going to be someone running faster or lifting heavier weights

FITNESS MAGAZINE MODELS

Comparisons will frustrate you, especially when looking at sport and fitness magazines. While some people find these inspirational, for most it can be really disheartening to compare yourself to these very unrealistic images.

Remember: The models are airbrushed—yes, even the male ones—after photo-shoots with fantastic lighting to highlight muscles. Some are even dehydrated to the point where they would do anything for a sip of water. It is not a look that is sustainable, and in some cases it's not even healthy (despite the fact that they appear "healthy"). If you can, avoid these kinds of books, magazines, or images unless it truly is inspirational for you. Otherwise, focus on images and books that do not leave you comparing yourself to other people.

than you, and that is okay. Focus only on you and your fitness level, and what you are doing to improve it.

Also, try not to fall into the trap of comparing your current self to your old self. You may have been an athlete in your earlier years, or in a position where you could eat whatever you wanted without gaining weight. But you are not the same person today that you were even a year ago. Events in your life change you over time. You are a product of your experiences. Focusing on where you used to be is comparing apples to oranges. Even if you follow the program to a T and lose all the weight you wanted and more, you will still not be the person you used to be.

Forget the old glory days and start making new glory days for today and the future!

HOW THE PROGRAM WORKS

I have compiled 20 years of experience and education into the following chapters and divided the program into a format that is easy to follow and incorporate on a day-to-day basis. There are five phases: Foundation, Building, Intensify, Advanced, and Sustainability. Each phase contains a set of workouts and a series of nutrition habits to incorporate from week to week. For exercise, you will progress from adding 10,000 steps into your daily routines to a weekly fitness schedule with specific workouts that include instructions on how to complete the exercises and any equipment that is required to do so. (Don't worry—it's not a lot of equipment!) For nutrition, each phase consists of habits that you slowly integrate, one at a time, into your weekly nutrition game plan.

> Each new program addition is a small step forward and is intended to become a natural part of your lifestyle instead of acting as a temporary solution to a non-temporary problem.

While each step is meant to be completed in a two-week timespan, 80% compliance is required for each before you move on to the next one. It is therefore possible that you take several weeks to nail a habit (something my dad certainly faced once or twice) or to get all your required workouts in, and that is okay! Be patient with yourself. It is better to wait until the habit is fully formed before attempting to stack on another one.

> Do not skip ahead to next steps until you're able to achieve 80% compliance over the span of two weeks.

PDF DOWNLOADS

Each section of *Reality Fitness* includes several PDF downloads available online at www.realityfitnessbook.com. All your tracking forms and all your workouts can be found here. You can print them, bookmark them, or save the PDFs to your mobile device so they are readily available to you throughout the program.

ONLINE NUTRITION SUPPORT

If you are looking to have more accountability and guidance like my favourite dad had, specifically when it comes to your nutrition, then sign up for the online nutrition coaching program. The program follows the exact flow of the one in the book, but also includes the chance to connect directly with Angela deJong on a bi-weekly basis to touch base on your progress and to ask any questions you might have. The program runs at regular intervals throughout the year. See www.realityfitnessbook.com for more details.

REALITY FITNESS
FOUNDATION PHASE

WALK IT OFF!

TAKE 10,000 STEPS EVERY DAY

Foundation

FITNESS

REALITY FITNESS NUTRITION AND WORKOUT TRACKER

		Week:								
		Weight:								
	Phase		Mon	Tue	Wed	Thu	Fri	Sat	Sun	
	10,000 steps									
Notes:										

		Week:								
		Weight:								
			Mon	Tue	Wed	Thu	Fri	Sat	Sun	80%?

It is important to develop a fitness base before jumping into more complicated movement patterns, and walking is an excellent form of activity to do so. As a weight-bearing activity, it challenges your skeletal system and increases bone strength, which helps reduce the risk of osteoporosis. If you increase your pace, a brisk walk becomes an excellent form of cardiovascular exercise. Walking also aids in caloric burn, which supports weight loss.

The main goal of this phase is to develop a commitment to movement within your lifestyle simply through walking. Incorporating a daily walking routine will aid in better health, a smaller waistline, and a true feeling of accomplishment. If you can dedicate yourself to taking 10,000 steps each day, you will be mentally and physically ready to start adding in more challenging activities.

GAME PLAN

Take 10,000 steps every day.

Speed is not a factor; complete the steps as fast or slow as you need. Running, jogging, walking, or combinations of all three are acceptable. It is the completion of the task—not the intensity—that is most important. The steps do not have to be completed all at once. You can accumulate the steps throughout the day, but be precise! 9999 steps does not equal 10,000 steps. And of course: the more, the better. If you can walk more than 10,000 steps a day, do it!

Track your steps by marking the days with a checkmark (or with whatever mark floats your boat!) on the printable tracking sheet that you will find at the start of the first nutrition phase.

If you are currently unable to complete 10,000 steps per day, start with what you are capable of. The next day, challenge yourself to increase your count by 250-500 steps. As your endurance builds, you will eventually reach your 10,000 steps. Write down the number you get to each day on your calendar. Once you are able to complete 10,000 steps 12 days out of 14 days in a row, you're ready to move on to the next exercise phase.

WHY 10,000?

10,000 steps a day is a concept that started in Japan nearly 40 years ago to promote more walking and improved health and fitness. Several studies have since found that walking 10,000 steps a day has a huge impact on body fat and waist to hip ratio, even compared to a 6,000 step a day count.

Today, the average North American walks approximately 2,300 to 3,000 steps daily (about 1.5 miles). In comparison, researchers collected the step data of 98 Amish-American adults wearing pedometers and found that men took an average of 18,425 steps a day (women took 14,196 steps). When this information is compared to the 3,000 step average North American adults walk, it is easy to see why only 4% of Amish adults are obese versus 41% of the general North American population.

RECOMMENDATIONS FOR SUCCESS

PEDOMETERS

The only way to gauge success is to know precisely how many steps you have taken or kilometres you have covered. But counting 10,000 steps isn't easy, especially if you're not getting them in all at once. Purchasing a pedometer helps you to track the number of steps you take each day. A pedometer—those small devices that clip onto your clothing or that can be worn as a watch—approximates the number of steps you are taking each day. These devices range in price and can be found at most fitness stores or large scale shopping centres. It is not necessary to get a top of the line pedometer. Any price point will work for the purpose of this exercise phase.

If you prefer to not purchase a pedometer, track your progress using distance as your guide. Eight kilometres (or five miles) is approximately equivalent to 10,000 steps. Measure your distance out in advance—Google Maps is great for this—so that you can be as precise as possible.

The only disadvantage to not having a pedometer is that you will not be granted credit for the steps taken outside of your distance tracking during the day. With a pedometer you are granted credit toward your 10,000 steps all day long as you move around. Without the pedometer you have to measure your distance out in advance, and the steps you take walking around throughout the day (to and from your vehicle, to and from your office during a coffee break, etc.) won't count.

Remember: Precision is key!

WHAT TO WEAR

Purchase comfortable shoes to support your hips, knees, and back, especially if you'll be getting all your steps in one shot. No one shoe is perfect for everyone. If you are able to find a pair of shoes that feel good on your feet, do not cause rubbing or blisters, and offer a little bit of cushioning for the soles of your feet, these will be great for your walking routine. Dress shoes or flip flops are not recommended for long walks as these tend to make your feet, ankles, and calf muscles sore after a while.

STAY HYDRATED

Take water with you to stay hydrated, and remember to stay hydrated throughout the day. A body that is dehydrated often feels more stiff and tired during and after exercise because muscles and cartilage require fluid to stay soft. Dehydration, especially during activity, can also lead to weakness, fatigue, dizziness, and electrolyte imbalance.

I had been asking Ang for a workout plan to follow for a while to help me get into better shape, but I never planned for 10,000 steps to be my starting point. That almost seemed too easy! I had a lot of questions. Why on earth would she pick a random number like 10,000? How do I even go about tracking that? Do I have to start counting every time I move? How long is this going to take me each day? Is walking seriously going to be enough to help me get fit? And where the hell am I going to walk? Ang assured me that this walking program would help me develop a regular fitness routine. Essentially, if I could make the time to walk in my day, I could make the time to add in workouts later on. Okay, I get it. This wasn't JUST about walking; it was about making movement a priority. So I put on my running shoes, stepped outside, walked my fat ass right past the SUV, and kept going.

I purchased a pedometer to track my steps and found it easy to use. In my mind, maybe too easy to use, which made me question its accuracy. And I most certainly wasn't doing any extra, damn it! I tested it for the first day of the challenge by counting the steps off in my head and comparing it to the little device. I used the "notes" app on my phone and gave myself a 1 for every 100 steps I counted. To my surprise, it was very close. (Or maybe my count was very close to its more accurate count.) Anyway, it was close enough that I trusted I did not have to count after day one. I felt confident I was getting credit for the effort I was putting in, and bonus: I no longer looked crazy watching my feet and counting milestone numbers out loud while I walked.

A pedometer really identifies how much walking and general movement you do in a day. I was surprised as to how little I was actually moving prior to this challenge.

> I thought I was moving a lot during the day, but the pedometer told me different.

So a pedometer is a very cool device that sure keeps you accountable. A pedometer is also a very annoying device that keeps you accountable. My first day out walking I had no idea how far I would have to go to see that magic number on my new device. Turns out it was a long freaking way! I thought maybe Ang had added an extra zero in there, and I was just over achieving the first day. I was disappointed to discover the news that no, a mistake was not made. I was indeed expected to walk for about an hour and fifteen minutes every day in order to pass my first fitness challenge. After a few days I suggested to Ang that perhaps this was a bit too aggressive of a goal for someone just starting out. Who has this kind of time? She told me that this is the suggested *minimum* amount of walking activity for heart health. She also said that this was the easy part.

> If I was not committed to taking 10,000 steps each day, I was likely not ready for real change.

That hit home for me. If I was already making excuses for this, then how was I going to incorporate other changes week after week? I had to change my attitude about it and figure out a way to make walking 10,000 steps part of my daily routine. So I hunkered down and worked out a way to get in all those damn steps.

On the days that I was travelling, I spent as much time as possible walking back and forth in the airport terminal to get steps in before I had to sit on the plane. I would switch the arm that dragged my bag behind me every ten minutes to even out the tension on each side to make it feel like an arm workout too! I know, that sounds totally ridiculous, and I wish I could say Ang told me to do it, but it was my stupid idea. What was happening to me? Why was I thinking about making this more challenging? I was impressed with how many steps I could get in—sometimes all 10,000 steps if I was waiting for an international flight. It felt good! In the past I would have just sat and waited, but now I was doing something productive. Once I got to the hotel I would fit in any missing steps by either walking outside to a restaurant or on the treadmill in the gym. If these were not options, I would pace myself and walk up and down the stairs of the hotel building to get my credits. This was not my favourite option because it was a lot more work, but at least it helped me get to my 10,000. (And yes, it would have been easier to pace the halls, but at the hours I was fitting this in I didn't want to disturb anyone's sleep.)

Before starting my fitness plans, I had booked a trip to Vegas to hang out with the boys, and it landed in my 10,000 steps phase. What happens in Vegas normally stays in Vegas, but in this case I'm actually *proud* of what I did, so I'll share my story. Well, some of the story. I'm not going to tell you *everything* that happened there.

I had made a promise to myself, and I was not going to break it. I was just getting started with the system, and I wasn't going to make excuses already. But the majority of the time we'd be sitting at a poker table or on a bar stool somewhere (drinking water, of course). I realized that if I was going to complete the 10,000 step challenge, I was going to have to either leave the poker table during the day or get up early to walk.

Not wanting to miss out on anything with the boys, I opted for the early morning walks. With the work schedule I kept, I was used to very little sleep, so every night (or morning, rather) after finishing up at the poker table, I made my way back to the room, put on my workout gear, and headed down to the gym to complete my 10,000 steps as planned. All the while the rest of the boys were asleep! Then I would go back up to the room for a quick shower and a nap before doing it all over again.

Can you believe it was $25 to use the fitness centre at the hotel? I could have bet that at the poker table, but instead I used it to sweat on a moving belt. It was happening. . . I was acting like Ang! Even the boys were impressed with my dedication. I don't think they believed I was going to do it, and believe me—there were many times that trip when I wanted to talk myself out of it. The walks felt long and more difficult than usual (maybe it was from being awake for 22 hours, or maybe it was because of the "water" I was drinking all night). But I was pretty pleased with myself for making the effort. It felt good to prove those guys wrong!

Back home I started to find it easier to fit the steps in. Often I would just go out walking for an hour and made this my exercise routine for the day. I preferred to get the walking over with all at once. Any extra steps after my 10,000 were just bonus points, in my mind. I did have to make changes in my regular schedule to have the time to do this, but somehow I was managing to still complete the other tasks on my agenda anyway. It just required prioritization of some tasks and boundaries for others. I was beginning to realize I had had the time all along, I was just choosing to use it for other things.

I liked having a number to focus on. 10,000 steps meant success, plain and simple.

It felt good to complete my challenge each day. By the end of the two weeks, I realized this was actually do-able and not nearly as difficult as I imagined. Time consuming? Yes. But physically hard for an able bodied person? No. My legs, hips, and lower back were definitely feeling the new activity, but I was finding it easier and easier. I managed to not go a single day without seeing at least 10,000 steps. It became a little game that kept myself challenged and motivated. That said, after fourteen consecutive days of completion, I lost zero weight! I was disappointed and complained to Ang about it. She explained to me that this is the reality of true fitness and of making changes that would last for life, not just for a few weeks. Fair enough. I was not a gym guy—and the idea of working out was a little scary—but I was ready to ramp it up! I promised to give it my all in the next phase of exercise. I had no idea what was about to come. I should have revelled in the walking-only days.

TERRY'S TIPS

1. Complete as many steps as possible early in the day. It's not fun to find that at 10:00 p.m. you still have 4000 steps to complete, trust me!

2. Buy two pairs of shoes that are different. I found that alternating my shoes every now and then helped reduce blisters and sore feet.

3. Get more steps in everywhere! Park as far away from the grocery store, bank, or work as your can so you have to walk farther. (I used to do this so I could have a cigarette between the car and the store. Now I do it for fitness!) Walk around the house or around your office when you are talking on the phone. It is amazing how many steps you get in doing this! Even walking around the house while brushing your teeth can get ya an extra 250 steps.

4. Do 'em all at once! I found it better to do most or all of the steps in one bout of walking, and then any extra walking I did was a bonus. This routine really helped me later on to find the time to fit in my workouts because the time was already carved out in my schedule. If you find a route that you make your routine track, it can be comforting and can motivate you to walk just a bit faster once you get going. You will have an idea of how long it takes to walk to certain landmarks. Each day you can challenge yourself to make it to those landmarks just a bit quicker to increase your intensity.

5. Create a music playlist that gets you through your distance. For me, 10,000 steps worked out to give or take twelve songs. The music was motivating and helped the time pass quickly.

BOTTOMS UP

DRINK THREE LITRES OF WATER A DAY

1

NUTRITION

REALITY FITNESS NUTRITION AND WORKOUT TRACKER

	Week:							Week:						
	Weight:							Weight:						
Phase	Mon	Tue	Wed	Thu	Fri	Sat	Sun	Mon	Tue	Wed	Thu	Fri	Sat	Sun
N1: 3L Water														
														80%?
10,000 steps														
Notes:														

Water makes up 70-75% of your total body weight; approximately 90% of your blood is made of it. Most of us are aware that drinking water is good for us, but why is it good for us? Well, outside of filling your stomach so you feel full and potentially eat less, water helps you:

- maintain your body temperature,
- metabolize body fat (that's right, it helps you lose weight!),
- digest food,
- lubricate and cushion your organs,
- transport nutrients to your cells, and
- flush toxins from your body.

GAME PLAN

Drink a minimum of three litres of water each day.

Other zero-calorie beverages are acceptable, such as naturally flavoured water, herbal and decaffeinated teas (hot or cold), and sugar-free/aspartame-free bottled beverages. However, this step is most effective when you stick to pure H_2O.

Avoid or limit beverages such as coffee, juice (even freshly squeezed), milk, sodas or other sugary beverages, diet sodas, and alcohol. For overall health it is best to avoid artificial chemical sweeteners such as sucralose and aspartame. Also avoid sports drinks, as these are high in calories and sugar content. You will notice there is often sugar hidden in most packaged beverages. You are not being challenged to omit these beverages completely, but be cognizant of how much you are having, as these eventually will be limited.

Sparkling/carbonated water is also an acceptable option for attaining your three litres a day goal. There are several soda-water makers on the market that do an excellent job of carbonating water. Be careful, though. Drinking three litres a day of carbonated water can lead to more gaseous consequences!

> With the addition of the water, the volume of other beverages you could consume will naturally decrease.

When it is hot or you are exercising more, you may find you're drinking more than three litres a day. This is 100% okay, and it's a good idea to drink more if you still feel thirsty due to the activity or weather. Yes, you might end up in the washroom more often, but your body will eventually get used to all the extra liquid and you'll find you're not rushing to the bathroom quite as frequently.

WATER, HEALTH, AND FAT

Drinking water is the easiest way to ensure you are keeping your body hydrated and optimizing your kidney and liver function. If you are not getting enough water, your body reacts by pulling it from other places, including your blood. This causes the closing of some smaller vessels (capillaries), making your blood thicker, more susceptible to clotting, and harder to pump through your system. This can have serious implications in hypertension, high cholesterol, and heart disease. Recent studies have also linked the lack of proper hydration to headaches, arthritis, heartburn, and decreased energy.

> In fact, a 2% water loss surrounding the cells in your body can result in a near 20% decrease in energy levels!

Water is also an essential component to proper kidney and liver function. If these organs are not working properly it can promote fat storage, making it difficult to lose weight. Without enough water, extra amounts of glucose can remain in the bloodstream until reaching the liver. This state of dehydration promotes extra glucose to be stored as fat. Dehydration causes your body to take water from inside cells, including fat cells, in an effort to compensate. Less water in your fat cells means less mobilization of fat for energy.

Dehydration can reduce your metabolism by 1/3!

Your muscles are calorie-burning machines and are made up of approximately 70% water. If they are even slightly dehydrated they will be unable to generate maximum energy, which reduces the number of calories you burn every minute of the day.

The kidneys are responsible for filtering ingested water as well as toxins, wastes, and salts out of the bloodstream. A lack of water in the body inhibits the kidneys from functioning properly, so the liver has to step up to the plate. As a result, the liver is occupied with helping the kidneys and therefore cannot perform one of its own jobs—metabolizing fat. A stressed liver results in less fat loss. Bottom line: if you are trying to decrease the amount of fat on your body, hydration is key, which is why drinking three litres a day is the first nutrition step in the program.

WATER AND EXERCISE

It's been stated quite obviously by now—water is important for overall health. Water is one of the most important components to a well-rounded nutrition program.

> A dehydrated body simply does not run as efficiently as it should, and this is especially true when you're exercising.

Proper hydration plays a major role in being able to contract your muscles fully, which aids in better muscle tone. It quickens muscle response and reduces muscle cramping so you have better overall performance in the gym and faster results. Being hydrated also helps you recover from exercise by keeping your muscles and joints soft, and aids in the mobilization of nutrients to your cells for better muscle development.

> Think of water as a natural optimizer that ensures you're getting the most of your efforts when it comes to your exercise (and your future nutrition phases too).

RECOMMENDATIONS FOR SUCCESS

DIVIDE YOUR DAY
Three litres can seem like a lot, but if you divide the day into sections it will go down as fast as the hours seem to go by. Drink a litre in the morning, a litre in the afternoon, and a litre in the evening. This way you don't get to ten at night with still two litres to go to reach your goal. Drinking water in this way also helps you to avoid needing the washroom more often throughout the day (and in the middle of the night).

WATER BOTTLES AND ELASTICS
To keep track of how much water you've had in a day, purchase a 1L water bottle and put three elastic bands around it. Each time you drink a bottle, take a band off.

IMPROVING TASTE
Not enjoying the taste of water is a common reason many people give for not drinking enough of it. There are many low to no-calorie ways to make water more palatable, though. Adding small bits of fruit and herbs to water can make the flavour more appealing and add variety. Here are some examples:

- Pomegranate seeds
- Mint and cucumber
- Basil and lime
- Lemon and or lime juice/wedges
- Watermelon and mint

- Cantaloupe and basil
- Pineapple
- Honeydew and mint
- Frozen raspberries and mint
- Orange slices

T-MAN'S STRAIGHT TALK

Well, already mentioned earlier in this crazy book about *moi* is that upon starting the program I had a slight issue with freshly squeezed juice consumption. Ha! Go figure, at the time I thought I was really doing my body good with all that fresh fruit.

Now I know that you can overdo anything, even healthy foods!

Along with the many (and I mean many) glasses of juice I was drinking to replace my cigarette cravings, I was also drinking about a litre of milk every two days. On top of that, I enjoyed a few pots of coffee throughout the day and the odd glass of wine or beer in the evenings. Basically, I did not eat much food and was getting most of my calories from bevies all day long!

When Ang told me my first nutrition challenge was to drink three litres of zero calorie beverages every day, I was a bit shocked! How does this help with nutrition? How on earth would this help me lose weight? I knew water was supposed to be good for you. I mean, all you hear is: "Drink this many glasses each day." But who can keep track of 8 or 10 or 12 or whatever new number they throw out at you each season? That's a lot of counting! So I never really followed the advice.

A major concern for me was: does coffee count as water? It turns out I was absolutely justified in being afraid of the answer.

I wasn't worried about the juice or the milk (the healthy stuff) or even the booze! It was the coffee that scared me the most. How was I going to drink all of my coffee and now all of this zero calorie shit in one day? Of course the point was to reduce and replace it. I told Ang I was on to her tactics, and she did not deny it!

The first day into the challenge I got myself a 1L bottle so I could easily start tracking my water. I had no idea how much water I was already drinking on top of all my other beverage consumption, but I did drink it throughout the day. To my pleasant surprise, I was already taking in almost two litres and had to add in only one more. Adding in the extra litre was a bit of effort, or at least I certainly had to pay attention so that I did not miss it. The extra fluid did seem to make me feel a little bit more full, and I was having less coffee because I did not have room for it (time-wise and also fullness wise). I was beginning to see why this might be an important challenge after all.

I certainly would not have guessed it when Ang originally presented me with this phase, but the water challenge was not very difficult for me to incorporate (not to brag or anything). I was already drinking lots of water before we started. Some days I was having even more than the three litres because I was extra thirsty with all the walking I was continuing to do outside to get my 10,000 steps.

I am glad I had the chance to focus on this habit, though, as it helped me realize what hydration feels like. I know this might not make any sense, but adding in even just that extra litre or so of water somehow made me feel more healthy and active. Focusing on water made me feel cleaner inside. I definitely felt healthier, less tired overall, and my mind felt less foggy. Later on in the phases I realized water was also helpful for keeping me full and reduced overeating too.

The biggest impact from increasing my water intake was the huge reduction in headaches. Before I began this process, I would get at least two headaches a week. Today, I can't even tell you if I have a bottle of painkillers in the medicine cabinet. It wasn't that a glass of water cured a headache if I got one; it was that being consistently hydrated prevented me from getting one in the first place. It is incredible how this has impacted my life, and I wasn't even all that bad with drinking water to begin with! I can't imagine what shape I would have been in prior if I had not been drinking any water.

My beverages now include mostly water, two cups of coffee (a huge decrease from the two pots I used to drink), a glass of juice, a glass or two of milk, and the odd celebratory beer after a game of golf.

> I know I am hydrated when my pee is clear. Maybe too much information, but it is a helpful tip!

Today I continue to incorporate three litres of water into my daily routine. For me, it is not hard to do. By mid-morning I have already had one litre, by mid-afternoon I've had two, and by supper I am finishing my third. Most of the time it's plain-old water, but sometimes I go with the fizzy stuff. Flavoured Perrier is calorie and aspartame-free, and the fizziness is refreshing and tasty. It's a nice option if you want something like soda but without the calories and chemicals. Plus, it kind of feels fancy! Don't tell anyone I said that, though.

TERRY'S TIPS

1. Don't guesstimate! Just like your steps, be precise. Guessing how much water you are drinking doesn't work. It is important to know exactly how much water you have had in a day so you can confidently say you completed the challenge. If you get into the habit of guessing now, the phases later on will be hard.

2. Drinking all your water late at night results in interrupted sleep! Drink more earlier, and sip throughout the day.

3. Carry a water bottle with you everywhere. I always set my water bottle next to my phone so I don't forget it. I don't get far without my phone, so this helped me keep the water top of mind.

4. Keep a big jug of water in your car. That way there are no excuses when you're on the road, as tempting as that Double Double may be. You can use the jug to refill your bottle.

5. Every time you sit down to eat, drink a cup of water before you start. This helps you get your water in throughout the day but also fills your stomach up a bit and helps you eat a smaller portion of food.

After all my success in walking more and adding more water to my days, I did not lose any weight. I know, not what you would expect, right? This was very frustrating, but I understood that I was setting the stage—getting my body functioning properly so that I could lose the weight down the line. For the first time in a very long time I felt like I was taking *real* action toward something better for myself. I wanted to see weight loss results eventually, but just accomplishing my challenges in these first couple of weeks made me confident that better things were coming. I was finally feeling like I might be able to do this. I just had to have the confidence in myself to keep going, and the trust in my favourite daughter that she knew what she was talking about.

REALITY FITNESS
BUILDING PHASE

IRON & INTERVALS

AN INTRODUCTION TO WEIGHT TRAINING AND INTERVAL TRAINING

Building

FITNESS

REALITY FITNESS ASSESSMENT TRACKING FORM

	BUILDING	INTENSIFY	ADVANCED	SUSTAINABILITY		
DATE OF ASSESSMENT						
TIME OF DAY						
BODY COMPOSITION						
Weight						
Neck						
Shoulders						
Chest						
Waist						
Hips						
Right Arm						
Right Leg						
CARDIOVASCULAR FITNESS						
1.5 mile run time						
OR						
1.0 mile walk time						
MUSCULAR ENDURANCE						
Squats (# in 1 minute)						
Pushups Off Toes (max #)						
OR						
Pushups Off Knees (max #)						
Plank off Elbows (max time)						
BALANCE						
Right Foot Hops (# in 1 min)						
Left Foot Hops (# in 1 min)						
OR						
Right Foot Standing (max time)						
Left Foot Standing (max time)						
NOTES						

Now that you have successfully incorporated activity into your day on a consistent basis, it's time to take things up a notch and push yourself even further toward your health and weight goals! This next phase of the program introduces you to weight training (yes, lifting weights), interval training (higher intensity exercise mixed with consistent rest periods), and circuit training (a mix of weight training and cardiovascular training). A gym membership is not required. All of these workouts can be completed in the comfort of your home with a few pieces of equipment that are suggested throughout the phases. In the appendix of this book (and in the online PDFs of the workouts found at www.realityfitnessbook.com) all of the exercises are described and paired with photos so you have guidance on how to perform them properly. All of your workouts are laid out in detail regarding how many repetitions and rounds of the exercises you are to complete, and how many times in the week you are expected to workout. It is presented this way so that you don't have to think about it. Just carve the time into your schedule and then mark it off on your checklist!

The objective of this six-week phase is to establish correct breathing and weight lifting form while introducing circuit training and interval training. You will use muscles you did not know existed! Some of the movements may feel unnatural or awkward, and that is okay. Take the time now to develop impeccable form so that in later phases your body can adapt.

Your endurance will be challenged, your balance will be tested, and your strength will be pushed. It can be intimidating at first, but within a few weeks your confidence will build. The movements will become easier with consistent practice week to week.

Remember: if this were easy, everyone would do it. Fitness and weight training are skills, and it will take time to master the exercises.

Don't be discouraged. Pay close attention to your technique, do the best that you can, and have fun with it! It can feel challenging or downright difficult and yet empowering at the same time. Bit-by-bit, though, you'll see progress.

GLOSSARY OF TERMS

The following words appear frequently throughout the program.

Reps: Short for repetition, this is the number of times you complete a movement. For example, if the workout asks for 12 reps of bicep curls, lift the weight 12 times.

Set: One round of the specified number of reps. Your workouts will require multiple sets or rounds of the exercises.

Series: A systemized compilation of exercises or grouping of exercises. Exercises are to be performed in the order they are listed, then repeated for the number of sets provided.

Weight: The amount of weight you are using to perform an exercise. Sometimes this is your body weight, and other times it will require additional resistance using dumbbells.

Light weight: Weight you can lift 15 times or more with ease. This type of weight is used during your Super Pump and Sweaty Interval workouts.

Moderate weight: Weight you can lift at least 10-12 times with the last two repetitions being a challenge but doable with proper form. This is the weight range used most often in this program.

Intervals: A form of exercise that involves a cycle of fast or intense movement for a specific amount of time followed by a rest period for a specific amount of time. Intervals are often timed in seconds or minutes and have multiple sets or rounds. This form of exercise is excellent for cardiovascular conditioning. It will come as no shock that your Sweaty Intervals are indeed interval exercises.

Circuits: A form of exercise that involves moving from one exercise to another to another, etc. with an allocated amount of time in which you are performing each one (usually in seconds or minutes). This form of exercise is great for muscular endurance and cardiovascular conditioning. Your Super Pump workouts are circuits.

DUMBBELLS AND PROPER FORM

Some exercises throughout this program use your own body weight for resistance, but other exercises incorporate dumbbells (mostly light to moderate weight). Adding weight with dumbbells helps to isolate the muscles and increases the effort to squeeze them. A lot of people get hung up on the amount of weight they are lifting, and yet what's more important when weight training is the time under tension for the muscle being activated and the quality of the contraction. More important is the time under tension for the muscle being activated and the quality of the contraction. In other words, the longer and harder you squeeze a muscle, the more reward for your efforts. Know that simply going through the motions of the exercises and completing the workout—particularly with dumbbells—is not enough to get the full benefit of your exercise. Technique is critical to success and also important for injury prevention. When lifting a weight (or performing an exercise without a weight) think about the muscles you are activating. Pay close attention to your form, the speed at which you are performing the exercise, and the amount of rest you take between each exercise. If you use momentum to lift your weight—be it your body weight or a dumbbell—you lose a lot of the benefit. A bicep curl without weight but with a strong contraction in the arm is more beneficial than a bicep curl with a heavy weight that was mostly just swung up with momentum or the use of other muscles to help it up.

Two 5 lbs. and 8 lbs. dumbbells are a great start for a lot of the exercises in this phase.

If you have more experience with weight training, take that into consideration when deciding how heavy to go. If you are able to complete all of the repetitions of an exercise with ease, increase the weight

THE MUSCLES OF THE BODY
The exercises in this phase and throughout the entire program incorporate all of the major muscle groups of the body.

Technical Term	Layman's Term
Gastrocnemius/soleus	Calves/lower legs
Quadriceps	Front of your upper legs
Hamstrings	Back of your upper legs
Gluteal muscles	Your buttocks
Trapezius	Your upper back
Latisimus dorsi	Your mid & lower back
Pectorals	Your chest
Deltoids	Your shoulders
Abdominals	Your core/stomach
Obliques	Side of your torso
Biceps	Front of your upper arm
Triceps	Back of your upper arm

you are lifting. The last two repetitions in a set should feel challenging to push through. If they are not, move to the next level of heavier dumbbells. Start each exercise with the recommended weight, though. Once you are immersed in the program, assess if you require heavier weights for a particular exercise or not.

> It is unsafe to increase intensity before you can execute all of the exercises with pristine form.

As you continue through the phases you will see that weight training is a skill. It requires practice. As your form/technique improves, so will your ability to increase the exercise intensity.

BREATHING DURING YOUR WORKOUTS

It sounds obvious that you need to breathe during your workouts, however it is common for individuals new to weight training to hold their breath as they concentrate on the movement patterns. Here are some tips and examples to add into your training as you become comfortable with the movements. (Note that the exercise descriptions appear in alphabetical order in Appendix B.)

1. Breathe OUT as you PULL a dumbbell up, and Breathe IN as you LOWER it down slowly.

Example A: For mid rows, breathe out as you pull the weights up toward your side, and breathe in as you slowly lower them.
Example B: For ball hamstring curls, breathe out as you pull the ball toward your buttocks, and breathe in as you extend your legs back out.

2.Breathe OUT as you PUSH a dumbbell, and Breathe IN as you lower it back slowly

Example A: For a shoulder press, breathe out as you push the weight up, and breathe in as you lower it down slowly.
Example B: For a bench press, breathe out as you push the weight up, and breathe in as you lower the weight down slowly.

3. Breathe IN as you LOWER your body weight down, and breathe OUT as you push your body weight up.

Example A: For squats, breathe in as you squat down, and then breathe out as you stand up.
Example B: For pushups, breathe in as you lower to the floor, and breathe out as you push yourself up.

> Breathing Rule of Thumb:
> Breathe OUT on the exertion portion of an exercise

For cardiovascular exercises, breathe as regular and steady as you can, and do your best to breathe in through your nose and out through your mouth. This helps regulate your breathing so it does not become erratic when the activity elevates to a high intensity as it does with exercises such as side-to-side jump lunges, burpees, or skipping.

For static (isometric) exercises (planks, for example), breathe as regular and steady as you can, and do your best to breathe in through your nose and out through your mouth. This helps to regulate your breathing and will give you a focus other than the burning sensation from the exercise!

TRACKING YOUR WORKOUTS

Keep track of your workouts on the provided tracking forms so you have a record of how many repetitions you completed, how many sets you completed, and what weight you used. This information is helpful for you to see your progress.

> Progress can feel slow or non-existent from time to time, so having your workouts documented helps highlight the changes that are actually happening.

My dad often put a small blurb on his sheet each day to describe how he felt. Eventually he began to notice that the challenging exercises became quite natural with practice. Having that concrete record to look back on gave him reassurance that he was indeed improving. For this reason you will find a comments section on your tracking sheets. If you find it helps, make a few notes about how you are feeling about an exercise or the workout overall in that moment.

START WITH AN ASSESSMENT

At the start of every exercise phase, complete a fitness assessment. This is marked in your sample calendars by A*. The assessment tracking form appears at the start of every new exercise phase and is also available at www.realityfitnessbook.com. The assessment covers everything from your weight, to waist-size, to how many times you can hop on your right foot in one minute. Completing the assessment gives you a great indication of your current fitness level and is an invaluable tool to see your progress as the weeks continue to pass.

> When you are "in-it" each and everyday, it's easy to lose sight of how far you've come. The fitness assessment will provide you with evidence that your hard work is paying off.

Each phase, assess yourself using the same format, in the same order to keep the process standardized. Be honest with yourself when you evaluate your performance. Make comments if necessary to highlight how you feel during a particular activity, and be accurate in your counting. Half pushups are not pushups.

THE WORKOUTS AND WORKOUT CALENDAR

For the purpose of this program our focus is on fat loss, muscular endurance, and building a little muscle in the process. In order to accomplish this, the program uses a combination of muscular strength, muscular endurance, and muscle hypertrophy (growth or building) repetition ranges.

   8-10 reps per set = muscle building + some strength gains
   10-12 reps per set = muscle building + some muscular endurance
   12-15 reps per set = muscular endurance + some muscle building

As you can see, there is some overlap between the repetition ranges. This is why it's beneficial to do a combination of these to maximize your fitness level. Pair these repetition ranges with fast-paced circuit training and interval training, and you have a fat burning, muscle-building extravaganza! To cover all your bases, the workouts are divided into three types: Killer (K), Super Pumps (SP), and Sweaty Intervals (SI).

For each phase you are provided with an example calendar of workouts (along with descriptions of each of the exercises within those workouts and a link to a handy PDF that you can print or pull up on your mobile device). You are not expected to follow the calendar exactly as written. Perhaps weekends are a great time for you to work-out, whereas Tuesdays are simply a no-go. This is not a problem. Print off your own calendar and write in your workouts to be on the days that work best for you (or pop the appointments into your digital calendar).

> Just ensure that you don't accidentally miss any workouts and that you complete the workouts *in the same order* as is written on the sample calendar.

WORKOUT COMPLIANCE

How do you know if you are ready to move on to the next exercise phase?

Perfect execution of a fitness plan is not necessary to see solid improvements in your fitness. However, 80% compliance to the program is important for you to progress at a safe rate. What does 80% look like? 11/14 days your 10,000 steps are met, in addition to any assessment day that is on your plan (never skip assessment day), and ¾ of the workouts per week (never skipping a Killer workout).

If you feel your technique still requires more time to perfect, despite meeting the 80% compliance to the program, please take more time in any particular phase before you move on. Anyone who begins this program will be at their own starting point. Just because the program suggests moving on does not mean that it is safe for everyone to do so. If you feel like an exercise or certain workout is still a real challenge (technique wise), take the time to master it before you progress. You will still get a great deal out of the workouts, and your body will thank you for the extra time. This might mean that you are progressing through the workouts and the nutrition habits out of sync with how they appear in this book, and that's okay. Eventually it will line back up.

DON'T FORGET TO WARM UP!

To prime your nervous system and prepare your muscles for movement, it is important to warm your body up before you do any cardiovascular activity or weight training. The warm-up is a way to get your head and body into the groove so no time is lost trying to work out kinks. You'll find a two part warm-up in Appendix A. The first part uses a foam roller to massage your muscles, allowing for increased blood flow to the tighter areas of your body. Once this is complete, a dynamic warm-up helps your body transition from a cold, static state to a warm, mobile state, and gently raises your heart rate. Dynamic movements help improve functional range of motion through the joints and increase blood supply to the muscles to prime your body for the workout you are about to start!

WORKOUT COOL-DOWN

Ensure you give yourself time for a cool-down after each of your workouts. It's the perfect time to rehydrate with some water and to have a short reflection on what you accomplished. How great do you feel after your workout is complete?

As opposed to the warm-up, the cool-down is used to bring your heart rate back to normal and to decrease your body temperature. Transitioning from running to walking is an example of cooling down. Taking a slow walk and then doing some light stretching or less vigorous foam rolling can also help decrease your heart rate.

BUILDING PHASE WORKOUTS

All right! Time to bring in the workouts for this phase. In the following set of weeks, continue to get in 10,000 steps per day, plus the workouts listed below. To move on to the next phase of exercise, you must complete a minimum of all your Killer workouts each week (so 3/4 of the workouts) and maintain 80% compliance to your 10,000 steps.

BUILDING PHASE SAMPLE CALENDAR

WEEK	MON	TUE	WED	THU	FRI	SAT	SUN
1	A*			K#1			
2	K #1			K #1			
3	K #2		K #1	SI #1			
4	K #1		K #2	SI #1	K #2		
5			K #2	SI #1	K #1		
6			K #2	SI #1	SP #1		

* While the days do not need to be exact, add the workouts *in this precise order* to your calendar.

Killer #1

Don't forget to warm up and cool down!
Take a 1 minute break in between each set.

Complete *2 sets of series one* and then *2 sets of series two.*

SERIES ONE
(COMPLETE 2 SETS OF FULL SERIES)

EXERCISE	REPS	WEIGHT
1 - Squats	12 reps	Light to Moderate
2 - Plank Off Forearms	30 seconds	Body Weight
3 - Lateral Raises with ¼ Lunge	10/side	Light Weight

SERIES TWO
(COMPLETE 2 SETS OF FULL SERIES)

EXERCISE	REPS	WEIGHT
1 - Shoulder Press	12 reps	Light to Moderate
2 - Alternating Back Lunge	12/side	Body Weight
3 - Pushups Off Knees	12 reps	Body Weight

Workout Complete!

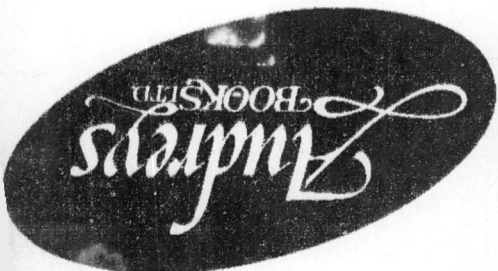

Fri Aug25-17 4:32pm
Acct: 148158 Inv: 636003 KN 01
Irene Serink
PO# 142810

Qty	Price	Disc	Total	Tax

9780995235106 Reality Fitness
| | 30.00 | 1 | 30.00 | a |

Subtotal	30.00
a GST 5%	1.50

Items 1	Total	31.50
Cash		4.50
Change		10.00

Killer #2

Don't forget to warm up and cool down!
Take a 1 minute break in between each set.

Complete *2 sets of series one* and then *2 sets of series two*.

SERIES ONE
(COMPLETE 2 SETS OF FULL SERIES)

EXERCISE	REPS	WEIGHT
1 - Stationary Lunge with Pulses	12 reps/side	Body Weight
2 - Lateral Shuffle	40 secs/side	Body Weight
3 - Bench Press Off Floor	12 reps	Moderate Weight

SERIES TWO
(COMPLETE 2 SETS OF FULL SERIES)

EXERCISE	REPS	WEIGHT
1 - Bilateral Mid Row	12 reps	Moderate Weight
2 - Walkouts	8 reps	Body Weight
3 - Toe Touches	8/side	Body Weight
4 - Side Plank Off Knees	30 secs/side	Body Weight

Workout Complete!

Super Pump #1

Don't forget to warm up and cool down!

Complete 2 sets of this series
with a 1 minute break in between each set.

EXERCISE	REPS	WEIGHT
1 - Bilateral Mid Row	30 seconds	Light to Moderate
2 - Pushups Off Knees	30 seconds	Body Weight
3 - Squats	30 seconds	Light to Moderate
4 - Lateral Shuffle	30 seconds/side	Body Weight
5 - Plank Off Forearms	30 seconds	Body Weight
6 - Jacks	30 seconds	Body Weight

Workout Complete!

Sweaty Intervals #1

Don't forget to warm up and cool down!

Do as many reps of each exercise as you can in each round.

Each round consists of 30 seconds of exercise followed by a 30 second break.

Go as FAST as you can without compromising good technique.

EXERCISE	ROUNDS	WEIGHT
1 - Jacks	4	Body Weight
2 - High Knees	4	Body Weight
3 - Weighted Punches	4	Light Weight

Workout Complete!

Before I go on about the workouts, let me tell you about the Fitness Assessment. Yup, you read that right. There is an assessment for this! I couldn't believe it either. Who on earth wants to go through a gruelling fitness test to find out what you already know—you're out of shape and a few .lbs over ideal. Ang explained that the "assessment" (A.K.A. The Brutal Test) would be helpful for me to use as a baseline comparator. I wasn't really buying it at the time.

The assessment is not easy, and how challenging some of the activities are might scare you or make you feel like crap about how far you have let yourself go. But it's your starting point—a reminder of why you need to make some changes. The assessment highlights areas where you are doing well and the areas that require improvement. For me, every area needed improvement at the start. I struggled to find something positive about the experience other than I completed it without dying.

As the weeks went on I was happy I followed through with the assessments. Knowing that there was another assessment right around the corner helped keep me motivated to get my workouts in. I referred back to my initial assessment at the start of every new exercise phase and went through the process again to compare my results. Sometimes my weight loss was not as good as I had hoped, but seeing improvements in my exercise performance (running faster, doing more repetitions, etc.) and a reduction in my measurements kept me motivated to continue. At least I knew something was changing for the better.

"The numbers don't lie," Ang told me, so I was diligent with my assessments and with recording my workouts to track my progress. It was surprising how quickly I could forget where I started or even what I had accomplished just the week prior. You'll see as the story continues that it is incredible what kind of strides I make in only a few weeks!

> My improvements were not a fluke; the proof was in the numbers, and I had the documentation to prove it.

Anyway, now into the story about the my workouts in the building phase. I admit I've wondered how open I should be when it comes to writing about the exercise components of this program and what it was like for me, especially in the first phase. I want to be honest about what it was like, but I also don't want to scare you or anyone else out of doing this either. Oh man . . . you are probably wanting to put this book down right now, aren't you? Before you do, let me go a little deeper first.

Let's just say that before I started I was pretty naïve to what lifting weights was all about. I grew up in the '70s—the days of Schwarzenegger and the movie *Pumping Iron*—so I had a distinct perspective on the matter. Lifting weights, in my mind, was for huge guys that grunted away in front of mirrors while the veins in their foreheads popped out. Although impressive, this was also a tad daunting and certainly not a motivator for me to slip on my (very short) shorts (again, it was the '70s) and visit a gym . . . ever.

Despite my impression of what it was like to be a weight lifter in the '70s, I kind of thought workouts at home would be fairly easy. I would be using much lighter weights than those guys at the gym. How hard could it be to curl your arm up a few times while holding a tiny dumbbell, take a break, and then do it again? It seemed like no big deal, all the effort would be just in getting around to it. Now, I believe a positive mindset is critical to success, but in this instance it was a bit of hindrance because I mentally prepared myself for an easy phase of training, and I had a very rude awakening on the first day.

It was December and the day of my first workout. Ang trained me in Louisiana from her gym in Canada via Skype. We weren't sure how well distance training would work, but it was surprisingly easy to do (logistically speaking, anyway).

Ang had emailed me the workout in advance, and I might as well have been reading the newspaper backwards. I had no clue what I was about to embark on.

Ang's mother, Diane, was joining me, so we set up our bedroom with two yoga mats, our exercise ball, and a few random dumbbells we found in the garage. I arranged the webcam so that Ang would be able to see both of us on her screen. The computer rang and I answered. There was my favourite daughter sporting a particularly big grin on her face . . . This did not sit well with me, and it was at that moment I realized I was going to have my ass kicked.

Before getting to the actual workout, we went through all of the exercises so I could practice the proper movements and form for them all. She demonstrated each of the exercises herself and then coached us through them verbally. I was surprised at how complicated some of them were. The squats in particular did not feel very natural. I kept wanting to bend down like I was about to pick up my golf ball from a hole. My knees bent overtop of my toes, but Ang said I had to have them over my ankles. Yet when I did the squat properly it felt like I was sticking my butt out so far behind me I was going to topple over. A few times I nearly did. Diane, on the other hand, seemed to breeze through the exercises. She had visited gyms in the past and, clearly, practice made a difference.

Once I had tried out all of the exercises one-by-one (and I highly suggest you do the same), we went through the actual workout. I truly have little recollection of the workout itself. All I remember is that I was breathing hard and couldn't stop ruminating about how out of shape I was. I was sweating so much! Huffing and puffing just lifting weights in my bedroom! This was not what I thought it would be like.

Ang, keeping track of our breaks, gave us one minute between each round to catch our breath. In order to buy myself more time every now and then, I would go "blow my nose in the bathroom." I'm sure Ang knew exactly what I was doing. Part of me wanted to figure out a way to procrastinate, but another part just wanted it to be done already!

I pushed through the exercise despite how much it burned—a feeling I had never felt before. Initially I thought something was wrong with my legs.

> It felt like I had Frank's Red Hot Sauce coursing through the veins in my thighs! Ang reassured me it was normal.

Returning from having to "check on the dog," I tried to bargain with her about what exercises we would do next. I offered to do more pushups if I could skip what would become my nemesis exercise . . . lunges. Of course, I did not win this battle. "The exercises that challenge you the most are the ones that will help you—" Ang started to say, but I rolled my eyes and my hearing blanked out while I reconciled the fact that I had no choice but to do the lunges.

Just 30 minutes later, Diane and I finished the Killer #1 workout. (The names of the workouts, by the way, are my little addition to the program.) I remember laying in the fetal position—half on the carpet, half on my mat—thinking about how gross it was to sweat on the floor. I tried to get up, but I was too tired to move.

The burning in my muscles subsided, and eventually my breathing went back to normal. All that was left was my sweaty, numb body.

> I was grateful it was over, but at the same time . . . I felt good.

Reflecting back to that moment motivates me to never fall to that place again. I cannot think of very many times when I felt that bad, physically. Exercise highlights your strengths, but also your weaknesses. I don't think we as a society like to have our weaknesses highlighted. Perhaps this is why we often want to opt for the activities we are good at and skip the ones that make us uncomfortable. If that is the case, it makes sense why so few people exercise on a regular basis. It is not easy.

By the end of the first six weeks I had mixed feelings about the exercise. I had gone through Killer #1 and 2, as well as the Super Pump #1 and the Sweaty Intervals #1 (which I liked because it added to the 10,000 steps that I still had to complete daily). The workouts were not getting easier, per se, but my tolerance was better. I felt stronger, healthier, and more confident about weight lifting. I had all that gym rat exercise lingo down pat, and I also learned that when exerting myself I have a tendency to swear . . . a lot. I knew I was ready to move on to the next exercise phase when I was able to complete all of my workouts with correct form and, in some cases, even with increased weight or repetitions. Transitioning to the next phase and changing the workouts made me nervous, though. It meant harder workouts and new movements to learn. Pushing through the discomfort was mentally taxing. I knew it was good for me, but that didn't mean I had to like it!

Despite my dedication to the exercise (I did not miss a single workout in six weeks), I lost only five pounds. The number was moving in the right direction, but I thought I would have lost much more weight considering how hard I was trying. I had to sit back and ask myself if I really gave it everything I had in those workouts. Weight training is not easy, but I believed I had. It became apparent to me how hard you actually have to work—both in exercising and in proper nutrition—to lose weight. Clearly exercising would either take a very long time to get the job done or simply just wouldn't be enough.

It is hard—if not impossible—to out-exercise a poor diet.

I was beginning to see how much effort it was to burn off my food choices. The discomfort of the exercise became a motivator to not eat certain foods because I knew what it was like to try and burn it off. Focusing on my food would be the big ticket to losing the weight, and the exercise was going to help me stay healthy and fit. With a bit of trepidation, I moved on to the Intensify Phase.

TERRY'S TIPS

1. Correct exercise technique is the most important component to success. Your body will naturally want to take the easy way out. Don't let it! The easy way out burns fewer calories.

2. The sooner in the day you do your workout, the less time it hangs over you, and the less likely you are to skip it.

3. There are no bad workouts. If you feel like you sucked the whole way through, focus on what you are doing well—even if it feels like the only thing you did well was attempting the workout in the first place. Nobody is good at everything right away.

4. Lunges are f*cking brutal. Just do them anyway. Trust me on that.

START YOUR DAY WITH A SUCCESS

EAT SOMETHING WITHIN SIXTY
MINUTES OF WAKING UP

2

NUTRITION

REALITY FITNESS NUTRITION AND WORKOUT TRACKER

	Week:								Week:							
	Weight:								Weight:							
Phase	Mon	Tue	Wed	Thu	Fri	Sat	Sun		Mon	Tue	Wed	Thu	Fri	Sat	Sun	80%?
N1: 3L Water																
N2: Breakfast																
10,000 steps																
Workouts																

Notes:

Breakfast is undoubtedly the most important weight loss meal of the day. And yet—though it's consuming rather than abstaining—many people find eating breakfast in the morning to be a hurdle.

The key to successful weight loss is using more calories than you consume. Your body uses calories 24 hours a day. How quickly your body uses those calories is called your metabolic rate. Your individual metabolic rate changes throughout the day and night, depending on certain factors such as when you last ate, what type of food you ate, whether you exercised (and at what intensity), and whether you were at rest or sleeping. The way to maximize the number of calories you use in a day is to maximize your metabolic rate. No, sleeping fewer hours each night won't help! One very effective way to do this, however, is to start incorporating breakfast.

Eating Breakfast = Increased Metabolism

Studies show a direct link between eating breakfast and successful weight loss. The moment you eat that first bite, your metabolism revs up, so the sooner in the morning you eat something—anything—the better. Eating in the morning has even been shown to be more effective for weight loss than a morning workout, for some. Not only is it a good nutrition habit itself, it naturally inspires other good nutrition habits. By eating something healthy in the morning, you'll find yourself eating fewer calories throughout the day, and you'll be more inclined to eat foods that are healthier for you.

GAME PLAN

Eat breakfast within one hour of waking up.

Yup. That's it. Break the fast . . . with anything. What you eat is not the focus of this phase, the simple act of eating is. Breakfast foods can range from a piece of fruit to scrambled eggs. Oatmeal packets, toast with peanut butter, or a small cup of yogurt are quick and easy morning fixes. Even if it's just a small handful of nuts, eating anything will make a difference.

> Maybe you're not a fan of breakfast foods, and that's okay. Try different food options, "breakfast" or otherwise, until something clicks.

If you want to have a chicken wrap for breakfast, great! Have a chicken wrap. A bowl of soup? Sure, why not? Bear in mind that later in the program you'll be encouraged to stick to healthier choices like whole grains, protein, and less processed foods, but for now the goal is simply to put something in your stomach first thing to kick start your day and metabolism.

SKIPPING BREAKFAST – THE BARRIERS

Some people think that skipping breakfast will help them lose weight. It won't. If you skip breakfast, you lose the benefit of elevating your metabolism right away, and then you are burdened with a lower metabolic rate and lower blood sugar levels, which inevitably leads to lethargy and overeating later on (and likely unhealthier choices due to fatigue).

> For this program you must dedicate time not just to working out but also to eating healthy, and eating healthy includes eating breakfast.

This phase is crucial for weight loss. Losing weight is so much easier with the additional metabolic boost in the morning. It is well worth the time and effort to experiment with breakfast alternatives until you find something you can eat first thing in the morning. Here are a couple other barriers to eating breakfast, and tips for how to bust through them.

BARRIER # 1 I DON'T HAVE TIME

Lack of time cannot be an excuse for not making breakfast a priority. To save on time, consider packing a breakfast snack in your bag or car to eat on the go—a small bag of nuts, a breakfast shake, or a piece of fruit. If you'd still prefer to eat at home, prepare your breakfast the night before at the same time as you prepare your lunch.

BARRIER #2 I'M NOT HUNGRY IN THE MORNING

If you find you are not hungry in the morning, it is likely that you are overeating at night. When you eat breakfast, you are less likely to overeat at lunch and dinner. Your body will have more energy, and you will automatically burn more calories simply because you have to use energy to metabolize the food you ate early on. If you don't feel hungry in the morning, slowly shift from eating lots of food at night to a little food each morning to offset what you eat in the evening. As your portions throughout the day even out, you'll eventually wake up feeling a little bit hungry.

SMOOTHIES

A smoothie is a great way to start integrating breakfast into your routine. Here are a few favourite morning smoothie combos.

The Green Monster
1 c baby spinach
½ banana
1 carrot (peeled and chopped)
⅔ c plain greek yogurt
⅔ c ice
1 tbsp honey

Banana Oat Shake
½ banana
⅛ c rolled oats
¼ c plain greek yogurt
1 tbsp almond butter
⅛ tsp vanilla extract
 pinch of cinnamon

Mocha Smoothie
½ banana
1 c chilled coffee
½ c almond milk
1 scoop chocolate protein powder
1 tsp honey

Berry & Kale Smoothie
½ c kale
½ c blueberries
1 scoop vanilla protein powder
½ c unsweetened almond milk
2-3 ice cubes

It only took me a couple of weeks to get into the routine of drinking the three litres of water I needed a day, so Ang upped the ante and added in another nutrition step to help me move forward: eat something—anything—within sixty minutes of waking. And "waking" in this case meant at the first ring of the alarm. You don't still have sixty minutes to eat after finally getting out of bed five snoozes later.

> Now, I knew breakfast was supposed to be good for you, but I was not really interested in replacing my liquid breakfast (coffee) with food.

I was coming up with excuses left-right-and-centre after getting the news about this step. My mind started spinning with questions. What am I going to eat? Can I still have coffee? What if I am not hungry? If I start to eat more in the morning, won't I gain weight with all this extra food? How much time is this going to take? Do I have to do this everyday? Am I going to have to get up even earlier than I already do to cook?

Ang and I talked through all my questions, and I was left feeling better knowing that for breakfast I could eat whatever and however little I wanted for now, and my coffee was still okay too. All I needed to do to be compliant with the program was eat something small, even just a half a cup of food like 12 almonds and a piece of fruit with my coffee. (I know, I know. 12 seems like a random number, but Ang likes to get specific.) Ang suggested a smoothie, as often drinking something first thing in the morning is easier for people that are not already eating breakfast. I found this to be the case for me, so I gave smoothies a shot. It took about five minutes to make, and drinking it was more enjoyable to me than eating a full Grand Slam.

As time went on I began to get bored with smoothies everyday. Ang suggested oatmeal, omelettes, Greek yogurt, frittatas, and homemade breakfast bars, all of which I enjoyed and eventually even looked forward to most mornings.

Breakfast was tricky when I was travelling for work, though. At this point in the program I was often waking up at 3:30 a.m. (yes, you read that right) to get started with my day, which meant I needed to eat by 4:30 a.m. The restaurants weren't open, so in order to eat early enough I started packing my own food. I would bring my small blender with me from home and then quickly visit a supermarket on my way from the airport to the hotel to get smoothie ingredients I could keep in the minibar fridge. This did become a bit too complicated, especially when travelling to Europe, as nothing was open. So, I discovered oatmeal packets that I could easily pack and add hot water to from the coffee maker in the room. Ang of course mentioned that this was not nearly as healthy as the smoothies, but at least I was eating within the sixty minutes. Sometimes we have to pick our battles. I made up for it with healthier options when I got home from my work trips.

Perfection is not attainable, we just have to do the best that we can with the circumstances we have.

Once I had made breakfast a part of my daily routine, I noticed a few big changes. The first was actually being hungry for breakfast in the mornings. Before this process I did not wake up wanting to eat something. Even the thought of food made me kind of nauseous. I now realize it was my overeating at night that led me to feeling still full in the morning. Once I reversed this by slowly incorporating a bit more food in the mornings, I began to eat less at dinner. It took me several weeks to get to that point, but I am happy I did it.

The second change I noticed was that I was beginning to feel hungry during the day. This alarmed me because I never used to feel hungry, even when I would go all day without eating. Usually that feeling didn't occur until around suppertime. I simply had no appetite, and coffee was my "food" of choice. I could not understand how eating breakfast (more food) would cause me to want to eat more later on in the day. I became concerned that with all this hunger I was going to eat too much and not lose weight. Ang explained that feeling hungry was a sign that my metabolism was finally speeding up again. It meant that I had burned off the food I had eaten, and my body was letting me know it was time to refuel. The very natural feeling of hunger is necessary in order to know when it is time to eat again. When you go long periods without eating, your body begins to adapt by saving as many calories as it can by slowing your metabolism down. This is not helpful if you want to lose weight. By adding in breakfast, I was reversing the storage-mode my body had been in for the past few years. I was finally seeing my metabolism work in my favour, not against me.

The third big change I noticed was my energy levels. Coffee used to make me feel alert and ready for the day, but that feeling faded fast.

Breakfast made me feel energetic and clear-headed instead of foggy, and it lasted for hours.

Don't be mistaken—I did not give up my coffee! I still drink it, but much less of it now. I feel so much more energetic during the day that I need less coffee in the afternoon to stay alert. Plus, with all the damn water I was drinking, where would I find the space for the extra coffee?

The fourth big change I noticed was that I was starting to lose a few pounds by eating a little more in the morning and a little less at night. Finally I was seeing some progress! This motivated me and made me realize that there was something to this breakfast thing after all.

TERRY'S TIPS

1. Create a list of breakfast options to choose from each day. This helps so you don't have to think so hard in the morning. With my list, I knew how much time each item would take to make, and I could more easily make it a part of my new routine in the morning. Make sure you have at least one option that you can eat at home and one option you can take to go. This eliminates the excuse of "no time to eat it." Me? My stay-at-home option was often a bowl of rice cereal with milk. My to-go option was either a smoothie or a container of yogurt with some nuts.

2. Eat a bit less at night (even if it is two or three bites less). Yes, this phase is about "revving up your metabolism" in the morning. But I think it is equally about eating less at night. The less full you are at night, the easier the breakfast becomes (at least that's what I found). I started to notice the shift from eating a huge meal at night and nothing at breakfast, to a bit less at dinner and few bites at breakfast, to eventually not over stuffing myself at supper and eating a meal size breakfast. I began to feel better and saw my weight creep down as the weeks went by.

3. Don't fill up on coffee before you eat. This can stifle your appetite. Plus, if you make it a rule that food is first, coffee becomes an instant reward!

THOSE LITTLE EXTRAS

*GRADUALLY DECREASING BUT DEFINITELY **NOT** ELIMINATING TREATS*

Part One

CELLIES

REALITY FITNESS NUTRITION AND WORKOUT TRACKER

	Week:								Week:							
	Weight:								Weight:							
Phase	Mon	Tue	Wed	Thu	Fri	Sat	Sun		Mon	Tue	Wed	Thu	Fri	Sat	Sun	80%?
N1: 3L Water																
N2: Breakfast																
10,000 steps																
Workouts																
Celly Countdown		5	4	3	2	1			5	4	3	2	1			

Notes:

At this point it is time to talk about the elephant in the room. I'm referring to those "little extras." These are the foods we love but feel guilty about when we eat. Maybe we even eat them in secret and then hide the evidence. Things like chips, chocolate, beer, ice cream . . . treats or party food. Foods that we all know are not healthy for us and that are certainly not going to be recommended in a fitness book, right? Think again, because I—believe it—encourage you to eat treats. It's important to enjoy special events in life (which are always accompanied by food!) or to enjoy foods you love every once in a while without feeling guilty, and this is where these foods fall into the program.

As mentioned, 100% compliance in this program is not necessary to see results. 80% is. By incorporating treats into your week, you will not only (with practice) learn to avoid that "all or nothing" mentality, but you won't feel deprived and can fully participate in life's celebrations without affecting your overall weight loss. You'll be confident in allowing yourself to indulge once in a while without letting it completely throw off everything you have worked so hard for.

You will never be asked to eliminate treats completely!

Many of you likely already incorporate treats into your diet and are (likely) including a few too many. Indeed, while you are allowed to eat treats during your week, you are going to be limiting the number you partake in. There will be four "Cellies" phases throughout this book. In each, you will learn to slowly decrease the number of treats you eat by limiting and planning ahead for your well-earned indulgences.

GAME PLAN

Limit your cellies to five per week.

First: what's a *celly*? This term comes from my dad who loves to golf and who especially loves the part where you drink beer afterward. One day he told me that he was off to have a "celly beer" (or rather a "celebratory beer") on the 19th hole after slashing it around on the golf course. And thus the term *celly* was born (for the purposes of this program, anyway). Why not make every treat in your life a celebration—a celly—of some kind?

Whether you're indulging in a beer, a doughnut, or a slice of cake, when it comes to your cellies, keep the portions reasonable, ideally between 150-200 calories. In most cases, the portion should fit into the palm of your hand.

BEWARE OF THE PROCESSED CELLY

Remember Lays Chips' old slogan: "Bet you can't eat just one"? Well, it's true because producers chemically engineer them to be nearly irresistible once you have that first taste. Cellies are 100% your decision as far as what you consume, but be aware that several processed goods are manufactured to trick your brain into thinking you could use a little more food, and a little bit more, and maybe just a bit more . . . and this can easily lead you down the path of a full-on binge. If you're choosing these types of foods, portion out what you're allowing yourself for your celly and then put the rest away in as inconvenient a location as possible.

It will be much easier to keep within the recommended serving size of a celly if you opt for more natural foods (think high quality chocolate or popcorn you pop yourself). These signal to the brain that you are eating food and, if eaten slowly, tell your body when it is satisfied.

A handful here, an extra scoop there . . . these actually make a difference. Ha! Thanks, Captain Obvious. That's what you are thinking right now, isn't it?

My initial reaction to this habit was: "I can have beer? Shit ya! Let me skip right over to my beer fridge right now." But then I took a moment to think about it and began to wonder how I could seriously eat or drink "bad" foods and beverages and keep losing weight. Believe me, I wanted to! But I was really worried it would derail me entirely and I would get fat and unhappy again.

My first week with this habit was a real tester. I was on holiday for a golf trip with the boys. Yeah, I know . . . a golf trip with the boys! And I was only allowed five cellies in the week? F*ck. Again, I had to really dig deep and decide what I wanted my life to look like. Old Terry wanted to pound back five or six rum and cokes along side some tasty nachos after the game, but New Terry was reminding me of how many friggin' lunges he had to do to get to where he was, and he did not want to waste all that work.

I would have to be strategic with my plan so I could still enjoy the trip without sacrificing all of my efforts. Here is what I did (and yes, it is sneaky . . . but it is technically compliant with the program). Ang is going to cringe when I reveal the loophole . . . but hey, I'm here to be honest. Plus, I know that if you follow the program to 80%, you will still see results, so I don't feel too guilty. Here were the rules for my one-week golf trip.

1. Follow all the phase requirements to 80% or more (which I did).

2. Do all of my workouts (which I did).

3. Plan my cellies based on our golf games (and just as an FYI . . . in this story, cellies will be booze most of the time).

And here's how the schedule panned out for the week.

Tuesday: I flew to Edmonton and skipped the cookies they offered on the airplane. That's one celly that's not worth it.

Wednesday (Game 1): I needed to get a head start on the matches, so no cellies (a.k.a. no beer).

Thursday (Game 2): I had planned for one beer, but I won and needed my head in the game to keep the winning streak going. So no celly.

Friday (Game 3): I was up two games, so again I had no cellies. I was on a roll and didn't want to mess it up.

Saturday (Game 4): I had one celebratory beer with dinner. I was still the winner, but I just couldn't resist this day!

Sunday (Game 5): It was the end of the week (as far as the program goes) and I still had four cellies left, so had all of them that evening (rum and cokes). But here is the loophole . . . The clock turned to midnight as our celebration kept going. It was now a new week, and I found myself with another five cellies. So I had all of those too! Hello, Captain Morgan! Turned out to be a pretty fun night. See how I made that work to my advantage? Ang is not happy right now. But it was a new week, so my celly allotment was replenished.

Monday (Game 6): Not that I had any left, but I was not in the mood for a celly . . . can't understand why. My head just hurt a lot! And let me tell you, my lunges felt even worse than ever on this day, but that party was worth it.

Tuesday: I flew home. Mission accomplished. Habits complied with, workouts completed, kicked ass on the course, and left the winner (again). 10 cellies—no more, no less—as planned. Boom, that's how it's done! You're welcome.

Outside of my golf trips and into real life, this crazy madness of Ang's began to make sense. Basically what she was saying was: keep my nutrition on point during all my meals and then add in a treat from time to time. This way I felt like I didn't have to deprive myself of some of the things I really loved like beer, wine, rum and coke, chicken wings, potato chips, and the odd ice cream. After all, this was going to be my life and I needed to make it realistic and doable for the long run. I felt that if I took certain things out I would inevitably go hog-wild one day and start binge eating. Clearly Ang was just setting up boundaries regarding these cellies. And good thing! If she hadn't, I would have had at least six to eight cellies a day on my golf trip. That would have really made my weight loss efforts suffer. Instead, I had a goal to stick to five cellies a week. That was much less than what I wanted, but it was still manageable. The awareness and management of the cellies was critical to my success. In the end, I got home after that golf trip a pound lighter, and I still had a great time! Lesson learned. You don't have to give it all up to see results.

TERRY'S TIPS

1. Pay attention! Don't scarf down your food; savour every moment of it. This goes both for your cellies and your usual snacks and meals. Sit down somewhere comfortable and really enjoy whatever it is you're putting in your mouth.

2. Leave the TV off when you're indulging in your celly. You don't even notice you are eating when you watch TV at the same time, and as soon as you are finished you are left unsatisfied because you weren't paying attention to what you were doing. You are then more likely to grab or crave more food because your brain hardly remembers eating any!

3. When temptation really comes a-knocking, use water to distract yourself from it. It's not typically hunger that drives you to eat more, its old habits like eating in front of the television. By keeping your hands and mouth busy with something (like water), you can save yourself from being tempted to pick at food you don't even really want or feel like eating.

4. Make those cellies worth it and have something you really love, not just something sweet or extra because it happens to be there. Make purposeful choices. In my case, that's easy . . . booze! Mmmmm, beer.

5. Choose cellies that take a while to consume. For example, a handful of M&Ms are gone in just a few minutes, but a couple cups of popcorn can last more than a quarter of an hour, if you let it. More time with that delicious goodness for approximately the same amount of calories.

EAT MORE TO LOSE MORE

EAT EVERY THREE TO FOUR HOURS

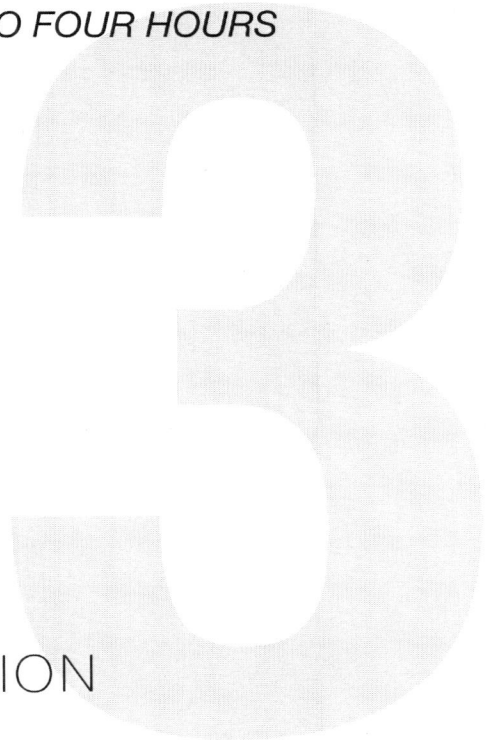

3

NUTRITION

REALITY FITNESS NUTRITION AND WORKOUT TRACKER

	Week:								Week:							
	Weight:								Weight:							
Phase	Mon	Tue	Wed	Thu	Fri	Sat	Sun		Mon	Tue	Wed	Thu	Fri	Sat	Sun	80%?
N1: 3L Water																
N2: Breakfast																
N3: Eat 3-4 hrs																
10,000 steps																
Workouts																
Celly Countdown		5	4	3	2	1				5	4	3	2	1			

Notes:

It may sound counter-intuitive, but to lose weight, eat more often. This phase of the program is again about increasing your body's metabolic rate, which happens every time you consume food because your body actually has to burn calories to digest it. In this way, eating and digesting food is almost like a mini workout for your body, minus the sweating! By eating more often, your fat-burning systems are working at a consistent pace, and this is how your metabolism is maintained and works best. Extreme highs and lows with food consumption during your day are not as effective for weight loss as a steady stream of moderate food intake all day long.

Many people, either purposely in an attempt lose weight or simply due to a lack of time throughout the day, skip meals. This is not an effective weight loss solution. Your body is designed for survival, and food is fuel. When you stop eating—when no fuel is entering the system—your body takes it as a sign that food is scarce; your metabolism slows down and sets to work preserving and storing (as fat) the energy it does consume instead of burning it at its usual pace. This is a helpful system if you are in a situation where you literally can't find food. But in today's modern world, if your aim is to lose weight, this survival system is a hindrance.

GAME PLAN

Eat something every three to four hours throughout the day.

Maintaining and even boosting your metabolism (a key to this entire program) is assisted by eating every three to four hours. When you are eating once or twice sporadically during the day, your brain might feel foggy, your energy and mood might be low, and your motivation might wane. By the end of the day, many people in this position are left feeling famished or "brain drained," so they eat a massive amount of food in the evening to make up for meals lost, and this has a whole slew of negative side effects including late-night lethargy and lack of motivation, then an uncomfortable sleep due to that over stuffed feeling or acid reflux. For some, a lack of hunger in the morning (due to overeating at night) often results in skipping breakfast, which starts the entire cycle all over again leading to weight gain over time.

> The every three to four hour timeframe is best because you are periodically revitalizing your body with a steady stream of (ideally nutritious) food energy, allowing you to live your life fully day in and day out.

Of course there are caveats to this phase. First, the point is to eat more often, not to eat more, more often. While we won't get too specific about portions just yet, ensure you're not eating full meals five times a day. Second, eating more often does not mean eating all the time. Whether or not you're able to keep up with tracking it all, you are likely to over-consume and take in too many calories. While you'll have consistent energy throughout the day, you'll still have an excess that will need to be stored as fat.

Over the course of the weeks in this phase, you might notice that you eat less at each sitting. You will also notice reduced hunger, headaches, fogginess, fatigue, agitation, and other low blood sugar symptoms because you're keeping your levels consistent all day long. Even better, your overall energy will increase day by day. By splitting meals and snacks up every three to four hours, you're providing your body and brain a steady stream of energy without flooding the system. Plus, you'll avoid getting to dinner every night feeling ready to eat your own arm off!

WHAT TO EAT

While what you eat throughout this phase is not the focus, eating a doughnut for every snack will also counter any of the positive effects of trying to better and maintain your metabolism. Sugary foods are converted to energy immediately and therefore provide energy to the body for only a short period of time—not long enough to keep your engine running. Inevitably, you'll feel hungry again and want more food, leading to overeating and more fat storage. Alternatively, healthy foods that have less sugar and more fibre provide a slow, steady flow of energy to the body. You'll feel fuller longer and be less likely to overeat. You'll have the energy you need to carry on with your day until the next meal or snack.

Pay attention to which foods keep you feeling full longer and which ones leave you feeling hungry within an hour. This information will help you in the coming weeks.

DEFINING "SNACK"

Eating every three to four hours is important, but if you overdo the snack (i.e. eat too large of snack) the purpose of the phase is lost. Remember, the point is to fuel your body with what it needs. Anything more than what it needs will be stored as fat. Here's a list of great snack options that will keep your engine firing without flooding the system.

- Pre-cut veggies with hummus for dipping
- A handful of nuts
- ½ cup unsweetened yogurt
- An apple with 1 tbsp of almond butter

As a general guideline, one handful of something is a perfect amount for a snack.

PREPARATION IS KEY

Asking someone to eat five times a day is a big request, especially for those who currently only make time for a meal once or twice a day. Eating this often is crucial to successful weight loss, but life is busy and it can be hard to pull ourselves out of whatever we're zoned in on for the sake of eating. If you go into the gym without a workout routine, you end up wandering around with little purpose. The same goes for eating. Have a game plan in terms of when and what you are going to eat for breakfasts, lunches, dinners, and snacks and then prepare everything you need ahead of time. You are more likely to eat a midday snack of cut-up veggies if all you need to do is open a bag and start munching. You might find initially that you are eating the same foods everyday, for every meal. This is okay for now. Work on getting into a rhythm first. Later we will discuss variety and food choices to help tweak your routines to keep things interesting.

ESTABLISH A REGULAR EATING SCHEDULE

Ideally we could listen to our bodies to know when to eat. The problem is that our busy way of life has put us out of tune with our bodies. The best way to prioritize eating and to ensure you're providing your body with what it needs—and not more—is to make an eating schedule. Schedules provide structure and force us to pay attention.

> Making the time to prioritize your eating benefits you in the long term and prevent you from storing fat like a caveman.

In a perfect world you would alternate between meals and snacks, but having two snacks in a row to meet the four-hour window is okay, as is two meals back to back if that's how your schedule works out. Avoid eating only snacks all day, though, and as stated once before, definitely do not eat a full meal every few hours. Regardless of how your schedule currently falls, use the opportunity presented in this phase to alter your schedule so that you can periodically take fifteen minutes to eat. Remember: you are eating to support your metabolism and to ensure you're getting enough food (and energy) throughout the day. In fact, when your eating habits and energy are at a consistent level, you're more likely to complete your workouts too.

EXAMPLES OF TYPICAL EATING SCHEDULES

Early Riser		Late Riser	
6 a.m.	Breakfast	9 a.m.	Breakfast
9 a.m.	Snack	Noon	Lunch
Noon	Lunch	4 p.m.	Snack
3 p.m.	Snack	7 p.m.	Dinner
7 p.m.	Dinner	10 p.m.	Snack

USE LISTS

Eating meals and snacks can be time consuming, never mind the time required to prepare those meals and snacks. And it becomes even more time consuming if you need to find/decide on a recipe, go to the grocery store to pick up ingredients, wash and prepare the ingredients, cook the meal, and then finally sit down to enjoy it. Having to do this each time you need a meal or snack would leave you with very little time in your day, but if you plan it out ahead of time using lists, you can consolidate the preparation time.

Lists can help make the tasks at hand easier, from knowing what you're going to eat to ensuring you have all the ingredients on-hand.

Pick a day and time to plan your week. If this is too long to plan ahead, go with two time-slots a week. Choose your recipes, list your ingredients, shop, prepare, and maybe even cook your meals and divvy up your snacks ahead of time. I know, it sounds like a lot of work! It may be that you set aside time on one day to plan, another day to shop, and another day to cook. Whatever it ends up being, having the plan is your key to success. Consider developing this planning routine as part of the challenge of this phase.

Lists can help you to plan and maintain good grocery habits. As you develop your meal repertoire and find favourites, you'll be able to keep a master grocery list for items you should always have on hand. Here are some helpful questions to ask yourself when preparing your weekly eating plan and grocery list.

- What does my schedule look like?
- What types of meals do I need to plan for?
- When and where will I be eating?
- Am I preparing meals for anyone else throughout the week?
- Any special events to incorporate into my plans (birthdays, holidays, etc.)?
- What's in season?
- What am I going to eat?

When Ang asked me to start eating three meals and two snacks every day I thought: Who the hell eats that many times a day? How am I gonna make time for all of that? Besides, I was trying to lose weight. How would eating more often help? I was very skeptical of this phase, but I knew Ang wouldn't ask me to do something that would make me fatter. Since incorporating breakfast into my routine, I was feeling good about the changes I had made. Plus, I was starting to see a smaller number on the scale, so I trusted her and gave it a shot.

I used to put off eating during the day until I just couldn't take it anymore, and then I would eat until I felt stuffed and tired and my belly protruded out, tempting me to unbutton my pants to alleviate the pressure! The only snack I was used to getting in during the day was coffee, and while I was eating breakfast consistently by this point in the program, it was still a decision I had to make every morning instead of an automatic habit.

> Going from eating once in the morning with a huge supper at night to eating every few hours was a huge change. It felt like I was eating all day long!

I was paranoid to eat too much during the day and gain more of a gut, so while I complied with the program by eating every three or four hours, I kept the amount of food to a much smaller amount than what I would normally eat in a sitting, just to be on the safe side. Ang assured me that my approach was totally reasonable and, in fact, preferable! It was a strange feeling to eat and then feel . . . nothing. The snacks never made me feel full. This was a totally different sensation, but it was better than my usual feeling of extreme hunger followed by feeling tired and like a hippo who can barely move.

I don't want to use my work schedule as an excuse, but I will say it made this regular-eating-routine thing very challenging. I had no life routine, never mind snack routine, and Ang was asking me to make one. Was a handful of nuts interrupting my day really going to make that much of a difference in my weight? (*Yes!* shouts Ang in the background.) Okay, fine. So I started bringing little bags of almonds with me to eat mid-morning. Turns out it wasn't so hard. It felt weird carrying food around—hell, I might as well have bought a purse to carry all the food in—and I felt even weirder when I had to pull food out in the middle of meetings. But you know what? No one really noticed or cared anyway. Actually, some of my colleagues even started doing the same thing once they saw me months later thin and trim!

Still, one of my biggest challenges with this phase was developing and maintaining the habit of eating on a consistent schedule. With all the meetings and jet setting I had to do, my lifestyle wasn't exactly suited to permanent routines, especially when I was constantly in different time zones and in different locations—planes, hotels, airports, conference rooms, restaurants—where the dining options were limited. Never mind all the work details that took up most of my mental space! Needless to say, I was not always focused on when I needed to eat. Thankfully I found using the calendar on my phone worked wonders. Yes, that's right—I said calendar. Not a timer or some other fancy app. For me, setting appointments to eat was another way to ensure that I remained accountable to myself. As long as I was prepared with some food on hand, I was able to keep to the schedule.

When it came to choosing what to eat, over time I learned which foods left me unsatisfied and hungry, and which ones kept hunger at bay until my next alarm went off. Eating a bag of chips made me want even more food right away, despite consuming a lot of them! When I switched the store-bought chips out for homemade chips (made with real potatoes—trust me, it's easier than it sounds), I didn't need to eat as many to feel satisfied. Ang explained that it was the ingredients. Real food with some nutritious value kept me feeling more satisfied than packaged and overly processed items did. Believe me, I *never once* thought of eating as an exact science. You learn quickly what kinds of foods keep you feeling full until your next meal and which ones you burn through faster.

HOMEMADE CHIPS
Use a mandolin chopper to slice some potatoes thinly, spray with olive oil and bake for 20 minutes, then broil each side for about 3 minutes to crisp up. Season any way you like!

In the end, I used Ang's recommendations of what kinds of foods and portions to eat for snacks: nuts, seeds, snack bars, boiled eggs, yogurt, and protein bars. As it turns out, my usual coffee consumption naturally declined because there wasn't enough space for it after a handful of almonds!

The preparation component is really the key to success in this phase.

Every morning I would plan or at least guesstimate when and where I would be at the times I was to eat next. If I was unsure, I would pack something to eat just in case. Most times that meant I was packing at least one snack and one meal, and I packed lots of extras when travelling. As long as I did not find myself without anything to eat every three to four hours (and the food was relatively healthy), I was doing okay.

I can't say I was perfect. I had a few moments when I was in meetings and got involved in conversation so much so that I forgot to eat my snack. In those cases, I just ate my next meal or had the snack as soon as I could. I knew the timing was not perfect, but I was doing a whole lot better than I used to! One thing I figured out quickly was that the type of snack I took to meetings also affected my compliance. Take it from me: opening up a baggie of two hard boiled eggs in the middle of a conference meeting is not welcomed by your colleagues! Taking less stinky options made me less self-conscious. It kept me more compliant with my snacks and more discreet!

It is not my intention to sound like it was easy for me to alter my life to fit in so many eating breaks. Once more of a routine was established, or rather when I simply got used to eating more frequently, the easier this step became. It took about three weeks to get it right, but once I did, I felt better. I stopped losing my words as often. I remembered names better. I was less irritable, less distracted, and as a result, I gained more confidence.

This step was as tough as the exercise, but not in a sweating and burning way! At first I was seeing only a slightly smaller number on the scale—not much change. At this point Ang reminded me that while the number wasn't going down, it also wasn't going up anymore. She was right! And while this phase alone does not necessarily help you lose a ton of weight, in conjunction with the following phase . . . magical things begin to happen.

SCENARIO QUIZ

Your only food options are what's available in a vending machine. It's all chips and chocolate. Is it better to: A) Skip the snack or B) Eat the chocolate bar?

Answer? A) Best to skip the snack. The sugar and fat in the available options offset any benefit of eating.

TERRY'S TIPS

1. Have pre-made snacks everywhere. With a phase like this one, convenience is not only helpful, it's darn right necessary! I kept pre-made snacks in my briefcase, in the car, in my travel carry on bag, at my office, and in my gym bag. That way if I forgot to bring a snack with me, or didn't have time to pack something, I had extras around to save me from going to the convenience store (which is limited in its options for healthy snacks) or the vending machine for a chocolate bar.

2. Prepare food for meals ahead of time. I like to wash and chop my veggies before they even make it to the fridge from the store. I also prepare and portion out the ingredients for my recipes in the coming days so that when it gets time to cook, there's less to do. Not only is this efficient in the eating department, it also saves a heck of a lot of time in the cleaning department too!

3. Technology can be helpful and fun. There's a ton of apps that can help. For me, I just set a notification on my phone's built-in calendar to remind me of when to eat. Every time I finished a meal or snack, I set a new event for three to four hours later (depending on my schedule) to notify me that it was time to eat again. For kicks (and in this program you need to take 'em where you can), I called my reminders things like "T-man's Shredding Snack" or "T-man's Energy Boost."

4. Don't forget about your water. If you find yourself getting fidgety or snacky before your timer has gone off, keep your hands and face preoccupied with that good ol' H2O.

HOW MUCH IS ENOUGH?

KEEP PORTIONS SMALL THROUGHOUT THE DAY

NUTRITION

REALITY FITNESS NUTRITION AND WORKOUT TRACKER

Week:								Week:							
Weight:								Weight:							
Phase	Mon	Tue	Wed	Thu	Fri	Sat	Sun	Mon	Tue	Wed	Thu	Fri	Sat	Sun	80%?
N1: 3L Water															
N2: Breakfast															
N3: Eat 3-4 hrs															
N4: Portions															
Workouts															
10,000 steps															
Celly Countdown	5	4	3	2	1			5	4	3	2	1			
Notes:															

This is the magic phase you've been waiting for. When it comes to food, your body only needs a little bit at a time to get all the energy it needs to function properly until your next snack or meal. The amount of food you eat at one time directly affects how much you store as fat. If you over consume food in one sitting (whether it be binge eating a bag of potato chips or grabbing a second pork chop at dinner), it automatically gets stored as fat unless you do some kind of activity to burn the extra calories off. Ultimately, weight loss is about using all of the energy in the food you eat and the beverages you drink, and then tapping into the excess energy that is on your body. That said, in order for the body to start using the excess fuel (fat stores), it must first be fed with good nutrition to coax the body to let go of it. This is why skipping meals does not work well for weight loss.

GAME PLAN

Eat the correct portion of food for meals and snacks.

& (yup, there's two in this one)

Drink only calorie-free beverages, with the exception of beverages that count as snacks (smoothies, milk).

The goal at every meal or snack is not to stuff yourself. You shouldn't need to loosen your belt! The goal is to provide your body with enough fuel to get you to your next fuelling point—to feel satisfied and energized, not bloated and tired.

Weight loss is just one of the benefits of reducing your portion sizes. You will find that you're less tired after you eat. Not to mention if you're eating less food, that means you're also buying less food, so you're saving money!

HOW MUCH FOOD IS ENOUGH FOOD?

Lay both of your hands down flat, palms up and pinkie fingers together, as if you were forming a plate. This is the space a meal should fill. For those that like to push the envelope, note that food should fit on two hands and pile up no higher than 1.5 inches. For most households, this is the size of a standard salad plate. For snacks, cup one hand. This is about the same size as ¼ cup of food, and this is the proper portion for a snack. When it comes to fruit, consider a single regular-sized piece of fruit a portion.

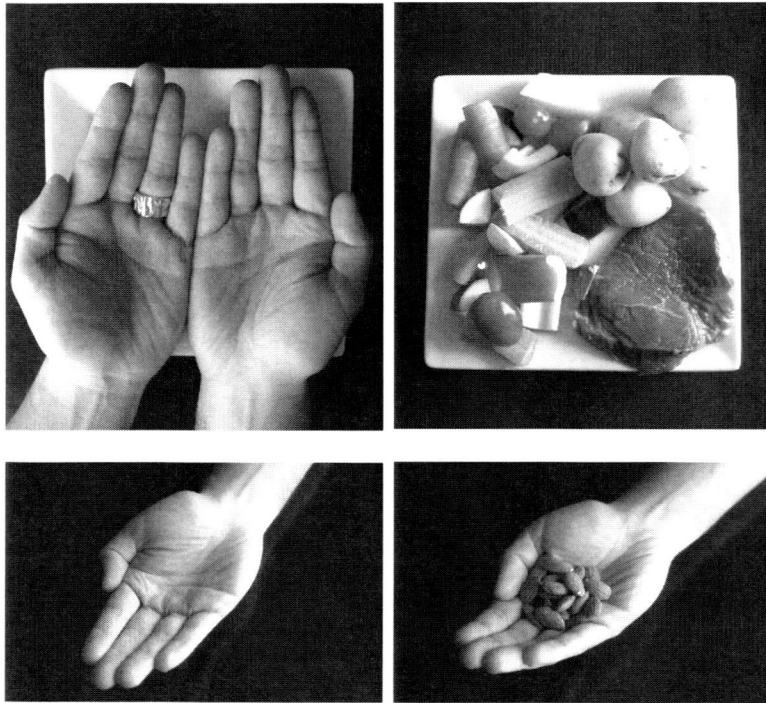

Don't worry. You will not go hungry.

There is often a bit of shock or even panic at this point. It doesn't look like a lot of food, and compared to what many eat throughout the day and at every meal, it is much less. But with weight loss, that is the point. After the last phase, you are already eating at regular intervals. In fact, you may have found that your portion sizes were already starting to get smaller.

BURNING FOOD OFF

The amount of exercise it takes to burn off a few extra bites can be quite shocking to people. For instance, two extra scoops of peanut butter on your sandwich is equivalent to about 160 calories. To burn off these extra calories you would have to run for about 20 minutes! Another example: maybe you are bored and feel like a little snack. You open up the pantry and grab a few handfuls of crackers. These equate to about 200 calories. It would require a 40-minute walk to burn these off. The point here is certainly not to demonize peanut butter or crackers but merely to highlight how easy it is to out-eat your exercise program. If you are going to eat, make the choice worth it rather than wasting it on a random handful of anything that's around. Think about your food choices before you ingest them and ask yourself: is it really worth it? Check out the following table that outlines some common food choices and the amount of work it takes to burn it off.

WHAT IT TAKES TO BURN

As a general rule, every 10 calories in a food item requires approximately 1 minute of activity to burn off. Note that these are just approximations. The values do not take into consideration gender, age, or weight and are simply meant to give you an idea of what it takes to burn off the calories in some popular foods.

Food (approx. # of calories)	Exercise to burn it
12 oz beer (195)	204 burpees
1 regular size chocolate bar (250)	70 minutes of walking @3.5 mph
1 plain doughnut (240)	88 minutes of crunches
2 slices of pepperoni pizza (625)	160 minutes of climbing stairs
¾ cup of ice cream (300)	30 minutes of circuit training
1 burger (320)	30 minutes of swimming @ moderate pace
6 honey garlic wings (960)	4 hours of golf (walking and carrying clubs)
21 oz pop (200)	54 minutes of lunges
1 cheeseburger and fries (690)	140 minutes on an elliptical
2 double-stuffed oreos (300)	70 minutes of weight lifting
1 small cinnamon bun (145)	28 minutes of jumping jacks
5 oz red wine (125)	30 minutes of weight training
1 coffee shop muffin (475)	120 minutes of housework
1 large popcorn with butter (1200)	90 minutes of jogging at 8 min/mile pace
1 slice of bacon (40)	43 pushups
1 hot dog (180)	55 minutes of consecutive burpees
1 dinner roll with butter (180)	18 sets of 20 pushups

I am not suggesting that you have to count calories. In fact, I am suggesting the opposite with this program, but it is helpful to have an idea of the calories in food to make an informed decision.

HOW FOOD MAKES YOU FEEL

When you started eating at regular intervals throughout the day, you were asked to pay attention to how different foods made you feel. Now is the time to focus on it even more.

> When you develop an awareness around what you eat
> —when you're paying attention—you derive more pleasure
> from your food. It even tastes better!

The type of food you eat is critical when it comes to how full or satisfied you are after eating a meal or snack. Pay attention! Questions like the following can help you figure out how your body responds to different foods.

- After eating that handful of veggies, how did you feel an hour later? Two hours later? Four hours later?
- When you opt for a chocolate-dipped granola bar, how long after eating it do you feel starved?
- When you are surprised at the sound of your alarm reminding you to eat again already and you are still not that hungry after your last snack, think back: what was it that you ate?
- Did you feel like you wanted to have "just a little bit more" after your last snack?
- After your meal are you feeling tired, bloated, energetic, or light? Do you feel better or worse?
- Do you feel guilty or proud after that last meal?

Each and every body reacts differently to different foods. Some feel energized after a slice of toast, others feel bloated. A banana might carry one person all the way through to their next meal, while another person might feel hungry again just an hour later.

A commonality is that processed and unhealthy foods leave you feeling hungry again sooner than non-processed foods.

While you aren't being asked to get specific just yet in your food choices, focusing on eating healthier options will enable you to feel satisfied and energized.

CUTTING CALORIC BEVERAGES

When we talk about portions, it means more than just what's on your plate. You must be aware of what you are consuming to make meaningful change, and those glasses and bottles of liquid are huge contributors to your overall consumption in the day. On average, a small latte or a can of pop equates to around 150 calories (about the same number of calories you should eat per snack). With just a few beverages, a person could consume just as many calories in liquid form as they do in eating food! While you need to be careful not to *out-eat* your exercise regime, you also need to be careful not to *out-drink* it. What does this mean?

From now on, opt for liquids that are zero calories.

Avoid sodas, fruit juices (even the freshly squeezed variety), milkshakes, flavoured coffee and tea drinks such as lattes and frappuccinos, and alcohol. Instead, stick to water (plain, flavoured, carbonated), black coffee (splashes of milk are acceptable), and green or herbal teas. Diet sodas are acceptable, too, although keep these to a minimum. They are not beneficial to your health in the long-term due to the aspartame.

The only exception to this is a smoothie as a meal (500 mL) or snack (250mL), milk as a snack (250 mL), or having a drink as a celly.

If the alarm bells are ringing for you right now, opt to start by switching out one caloric beverage with water each day. Get comfortable with this change and then switch out another. Once you've been successful in cutting out caloric beverages from your diet, along with controlling your portions of food, you'll be ready to move on to the next phase.

The day Ang asked me to lay my hands down flat on the table beside one another and observe, I thought she was going to perform some sort of magic trick. I waited for an explanation. What was I doing this for?

"This is how much food you should be eating in one meal," Ang explained.

"Minimum?" I asked, hopeful but fearing that probably wasn't the case.

"Maximum."

Fear confirmed.

I was eating at least twice this amount at every meal. If I cut it in half, I was going to starve to death! Was she trying to kill me?!

Despite my protests, it was clear that my current portions were not working in my favour, so I relented. Would I be starving? I might feel like it, but not literally.

> I would still get to eat every few hours. Maybe there would be some discomfort in between, but I would be able to deal with *that* discomfort better than I was currently dealing with not feeling comfortable in my own skin.

On day one of the new portion adjustment I had my breakfast on a salad-sized plate (rather than a full dinner plate) and was surprised to find that my food filled the entire surface area without going over. I was still eating about the same amount of food as before, it just appeared like I was eating more. I know it sounds crazy, especially because it was not as if I did not know what had changed, but the image of the full plate gave me a sense of satisfaction. After I finished breakfast, I felt content—not stuffed full, but content. Turns out my breakfast portions were pretty darn good to begin with.

I typically packed my lunch when I was working, and I found it was also fairly easy to stick with the smaller plate portion for lunches too. We have these glass containers that are nearly the same size as our salad plates. I use these and only these for measuring my lunch portions. I do not trust myself enough to not add a little extra scoop in containers that are bigger than they need to be, and eyeballing things is never an option! Most days, though, I typically ate a sandwich of some kind. And knowing that a sky-high sandwich was not in accordance with what I was supposed to be doing, I went with regular sized sandwich bread and no more than two or three fillers.

Funny, I used to be the guy that wouldn't even think about food. Now that my body was burning calories more steadily (i.e. my metabolism was working), I was hungry more often, and I actually desired food. I stopped needing to use my calendar to remind me when to snack because I could simply feel it. And when it was time for a snack, I kept my portion to one handful of something or a small glass of milk.

Dinner was the biggest challenge. In the past, I would have huge dinners—sometimes with seconds—and cleaned my plate, because not wasting food was ingrained in me as a kid.

> I was so used to filling my plate up in a heaping mound that when I looked at that little plate for the first time, it looked sort of sad.

I started the process by still heaping food onto my plate, but onto a little plate instead of a big one. Not ideal, but it was still less food, so this was progress. When the shock of this subsisted I began to heap a little less, and then a little less. Everyday I left a little less off my plate until the amount of food was in line with what Ang suggested. It took me a couple of weeks to get to this point.

At restaurants I would often stick to ordering an appetizer only. If I opted for an entrée, though, knowing the portions are massive compared to a puny salad plate, I would ask the serving staff to box half of my meal up before bringing anything to the table. That way I avoided being tempted to eat it all. Yes, I got funny looks from time to time, but it was the only way to make it easier for myself. I did not find I was successful when I had to leave food on my plate. It was just too easy to have an extra forkful, and then another, and then another, and then: Oh, well I might as well finish it now.

I cannot comment on this phase without mentioning the beverages that were eliminated. It never occurred to me how many extra calories I was getting just in the beverages I was drinking. I knew beer was probably not performance enhancing (although it sure seemed to help my dancing), but milk was not even on my radar as a contributing factor to my weight. Milk is healthy for you, I thought, and at three to five glasses a day, milk was an integral part of every meal I ate. I really, really, really did not want to ask Ang about it because I knew it was probably a bit of a cheat to have all of that in addition to my plate of food. Of course it's too much milk for one day and would not comply with the phase rules. I tried to make a case for it ("The calcium! I need the calcium!"), but Ang told me that by the time I was through this program, I'd be getting calcium through other sources in the foods I ate. Letting go of my milk habit was probably one of the hardest things I had to do in this entire system. Today, I only have a small glass of milk for a snack the odd time, though I still like to add it to my coffee daily—Ang knows that's a non-negotiable for me.

Breakfast, lunch, or dinner, I tried to make food last by eating slowly and actually paying attention to what it tasted like. This helped a bit, and I realized that I might have been overeating simply because I was going too fast. I was not actually that hungry, I was just used to eating a lot more food and wasn't giving my brain a chance to catch up to my body. I can admit that in the past after a huge meal the feeling of fullness and tiredness was front and centre. I just thought this was how everyone felt after they ate, and that was the goal: to be so full I felt like lying down and loosening my belt for relief! Today I have a completely different perspective.

> When I eat, the purpose is not to stuff in as much food as I can, the purpose is to satisfy me enough and carry me over to my next snack or meal.

Sticking to my decision of losing weight vs. falling into my old ways was very challenging, and I really felt it in this phase. Every now and then I'd feel like adding just a little more food to my plate. But that was an Old Terry habit, and what I had been doing was not working, plain and simple. In those moments of temptation I reminded myself that my old ways were what got me into this position, and the only way to get out was to make new decisions, which included eating less at each meal.

> For the record, I still eat quite a bit of food, just not all at once.

Knowing I can eat again in a few hours makes eating smaller portions satisfying. I don't feel like I am missing out. Even though the habit of wanting to eat more food is still there to this day, I resist the temptation to add extra to my already healthy portions because I know I don't really need it. If I overdo it and eat too much at a time, my body's only choice is to store the excess—that's the fancy way of saying adding it to my fat gut! And I work too damn hard in the gym to waste it on an extra portion of anything.

TERRY'S TIPS

1. Chew more, eat slowly. Before this phase I would still be chewing as I was adding the next bite to my mouth. Now I chew one mouthful, swallow, and then add more food. I know this sounds ridiculous, but I bet if you pay attention to how you are eating you'll find you're doing the same thing. Twenty minutes to eat your meal is ideal because your brain has a chance to catch up to your stomach to let you know when you are satisfied and have had enough food.

2. Eat foods that make your body feel full. I paid attention to what foods made me feel more full and satisfied vs. what foods made me feel hungry within an hour of eating them. I did my best to eat the foods that made me feel satisfied.

3. Never eat out of a container/package/box. It is too easy to underestimate the amount you're eating if you keep pulling bites from a package. Pour out a handful so you know you're not overdoing it.

4. Order small. If I were ever ordering an item that required a size selection, I always ordered a small to keep my portions in check. My idea was that ordering a small would equate to a smaller gut. This went for my cellies too.

5. Again, don't forget your water. If you are really wanting more food, rely on your water to keep your mouth and hands busy. I found that often it was just the habit of eating a lot at one sitting that was holding me back, not true hunger.

REALITY FITNESS
INTENSIFY PHASE

RAMP IT UP!

HEAVIER DUMBBELLS, STIFFER MUSCLES, AND MORE SWEAT

Intensify

FITNESS

REALITY FITNESS ASSESSMENT TRACKING FORM

	BUILDING	INTENSIFY	ADVANCED	SUSTAINABILITY		
DATE OF ASSESSMENT						
TIME OF DAY						
BODY COMPOSITION						
Weight						
Neck						
Shoulders						
Chest						
Waist						
Hips						
Right Arm						
Right Leg						
CARDIOVASCULAR FITNESS						
1.5 mile run time						
OR						
1.0 mile walk time						
MUSCULAR ENDURANCE						
Squats (# in 1 minute)						
Pushups Off Toes (max #)						
OR						
Pushups Off Knees (max #)						
Plank off Elbows (max time)						
BALANCE						
Right Foot Hops (# in 1 min)						
Left Foot Hops (# in 1 min)						
OR						
Right Foot Standing (max time)						
Left Foot Standing (max time)						
NOTES						

The next set of weeks is based on the building phase, with exercises that are slightly more advanced. While many movements are similar, some are completely new, and some now incorporate a balance or rotation component. Other exercises require an increase in the amount of body weight you are supporting or pushing (for example, going from pushups off the knees to pushups off the toes).

Outside of simply easing boredom, the variety in the exercise is important to keep your body guessing and helps to target as many muscle groups as possible, hence why we switch up the workouts every 4-6 weeks and do different types of workouts within those weeks. This approach reduces the risk of injury from overuse and hinders your body's ability to find the most efficient way to handle the exertion that you are placing on it (i.e. your body continues to burn just as many calories). By switching it up, your body cannot anticipate the stress and therefore must adapt to the changes, which in turn changes you—for the better—by making you stronger.

Despite using a lot of the same muscles you've been using for the last month, with these new workout routines you are likely to feel stiff and sore again for a while. Don't allow it to affect your form!

Remember that form is the most important aspect of proper exercise.

If you are unable to complete a full set properly, take a break for a minute and see if that helps you to regain the correct form. If not, complete as many repetitions as you can with good form, then move on to the next exercise.

Finally, you may be surprised at how the workouts, which seem simple on paper, can really get your cardio going and make you sweat. Any exercise that uses the large muscle groups—your legs, back, or chest—can really get your heart pumping, so know that it's normal to feel out of breath . . . they are a challenge. A big challenge!

INTENSIFY WORKOUTS

In the following set of weeks, continue to get in 10,000 steps per day, plus the workouts listed below. To move on to the next phase of exercise, you must complete a minimum of 3/4 of the workouts, and you cannot skip any Killer workouts. Don't forget to maintain 80% compliance with your 10,000 steps a day too. Adjust your calendar according to your schedule, but remember to keep all the workouts in the same order!

SAMPLE INTENSIFY WORKOUT CALENDAR

WEEK	MON	TUE	WED	THU	FRI	SAT	SUN
1	A*	SI #1		SI #2	K #3		
2	K #3	SI #1		SI #2	K# 3		
3	K #4	SI #1	K #3	SI #2	K# 4		
4	K #4	SI #1	K #3	SI #2	K #4		
5	SP #2	SI #1	K #4	SI #2	SP #2		
6	SP #2	SI #1	K #4	SI #2	SP #2		
* While the days do not need to be exact, add the workouts *in this precise order* to your calendar.							

Killer #3

Don't forget to warm up and cool down!
Take a 1 minute break in between each set.

Complete *2 sets of series one* and then *2 sets of series two*.

SERIES ONE
(COMPLETE 2 SETS OF FULL SERIES)

EXERCISE	REPS	WEIGHT
1 - Squat Press	12 reps	Moderate Weight
2 - Static Lunge w/ Weighted Arm Rotation	10/side	Light Weight
3 - Rear Delt Flys	12 reps	Light to Moderate Weight

SERIES TWO
(COMPLETE 2 SETS OF FULL SERIES)

EXERCISE	REPS	WEIGHT
1 - Single Leg Romanian Deadlifts	12/side	Moderate Weight
2 - Side Plank Off Toes	30 secs/side	Body Weight
3 - Side Lunges (Static)	12/side	Body Weight
4 - Surrenders	8/side	Light Weight

Workout Complete!

Killer #4

Don't forget to warm up and cool down!
Take a 1 minute break in between each set.

Complete *2 sets of series one* and then *2 sets of series two*.

SERIES ONE
(COMPLETE 2 SETS OF FULL SERIES)

EXERCISE	REPS	WEIGHT
1 - Front Squats	12 reps	Moderate Weight
2 - Alternating Mid Row	12/side	Moderate Weight
3 - Single Leg Lunge with Lateral Touch	10/side	Body Weight

SERIES TWO
(COMPLETE 2 SETS OF FULL SERIES)

EXERCISE	REPS	WEIGHT
1 - Pushups Off Toes	8-10 reps	Body Weight
2 - Back Lunges with Forward Kick	15/side	Body or Light Weight
3 - Lawnmower	12/side	Moderate Weight
4 - Pike/Plank	12 reps	Body Weight

Workout Complete!

Super Pump #2

Don't forget to warm up and cool down!

Complete 2 sets of this series
with a 1 minute break in between each set.

EXERCISE	REPS	WEIGHT
1 - Front Squats	30 secs	Light to Moderate Weight
2 - Side Lunges (Static)	30 secs/side	Light to Moderate Weight
3 - High Knees	30 secs	Body Weight
4 - Alternating Mid Row	30 secs	Light to Moderate Weight
5 - Side Plank Off Toes	30 secs/side	Body Weight
6 - Back Lunges with Forward Kick	30 secs/side	Body to Light Weight

Workout Complete!

Sweaty Intervals #1

Don't forget to warm up and cool down!
Do as many reps of each exercise as you can in each round.
Each round consists of 30 seconds of exercise followed by a 30 second break.

Go as FAST as you can without compromising good technique.

EXERCISE	ROUNDS	WEIGHT
1 - Jacks	4	Body Weight
2 - High Knees	4	Body Weight
3 - Weighted Punches	4	Light Weight

Workout Complete!

Sweaty Intervals #2

Don't forget to warm up and cool down!
Do as many reps of each exercise as you can in each round.
Each round consists of 30 seconds of exercise followed by a 30 second break.

Go as FAST as you can without compromising good technique.

EXERCISE	ROUNDS	WEIGHT
1 - Jacks	3	Body Weight
2 - High Knees	3	Body Weight
3 - Weighted Punches	3	Light Weight
4 - Wide Jump Squats/Low Jacks	4	Body Weight

Workout Complete!

If you are reading this, it must mean you survived the building phase. Congratulations! You may be feeling a mixture of emotions right now. Nervousness, excitement, exhaustion, empowerment, frustration, exhilaration . . . I know I felt all these things. It was overwhelming, for sure, but I continued to remind myself of how far I'd come. What a waste it would be to give up all the effort I had put in.

It would be awesome if I could tell you it got easier in this phase, but it is still pretty damn hard. I still had a lot of difficulty during the workouts. My legs and arms continued to burn, and everything just got more challenging overall. But there were some positives too. I seemed to pick up the movements a little better in this phase, perhaps because I had the practice earlier and maybe due to a bit of confidence I'd built up. Also, the routine of fitting in my workouts continued to get easier.

> I scheduled in my workouts and treated them just as I would any other appointment — damn near non-negotiable.

The odd time when work had to take priority, I suffered the consequence of having to do my workout at some god-forsaken hour. Eventually my workouts became as much of a priority as shaving and brushing my teeth!

My complaining and negotiating in the first phase did not seem to help my cause as I progressed. I was certain Ang put extra lunges into this phase just to piss me off. The single leg lunge with lateral touch was one of the most challenging exercises for me and continues to be. I struggled with my balance on this one, so Ang said it was okay to hold onto something to start. I didn't have a bench (as shown in the pictures), so I used the second step from the floor on our staircase and held onto the wall for support. The front leg was the one that was supposed to be doing all the work, but the back leg on the stair burned so bad!

> Trying to walk after this one made me look like a newborn goat taking its first wobbly steps, and I hadn't even had a beer!

Reading this it probably does not resonate right now, but don't you worry . . . it will. I was a sweaty mess by the time I finished the entire new Killer workout, but I was relieved to discover I no longer needed to crawl into the fetal position to recover. This was progress!

During the building phase I did most of my out-of-town workouts in my hotel room with the inflatable water weights Ang gave me for Father's Day. But some of the new exercises required heavier weight or new equipment, so it was time to cash in some of my built up confidence and venture to the hotel gym so I could fully execute the plan. This first trip to a gym was not what I expected. Right away it became apparent that the idea I had of gyms was incorrect all these years. It was not a room full of super muscular, veiny guys in tank tops.

> Most of the people in the gym were just like me . . . regular people trying to be a bit better one workout at a time, and surviving it.

During this phase I had another work trip that took me to France for ten days. I was unable to find a hotel that offered a fitness centre, so I packed my water weights again. This was definitely an opportunity for me to skip my workouts due to long workdays (some were more than 16 hours), and a real lack of space in my room. I could barely stretch out on the floor to perform a plank. I really wanted to just not do the program for that time period, but something was nagging me in the back of my mind. And for the first time, it wasn't Ang . . . it was me. This was a defining moment. Having a daughter who turned out to be a fitness trainer is definitely an advantage. Up until this time I relied on her to push me to keep going. She didn't always have to be there for my workouts or have to convince me to even do them, but I always had it in the back of my mind that I had to keep going so I did not let her down.

> But something had changed on this trip… now I too was holding myself accountable *to me*!

Was I doing my best? Yes. How would I feel physically if I didn't do my workout? Shitty. What were the alternatives to not working out anymore? Regaining the dozen or so pounds I had lost up to this point. How would I feel about myself if I just quit all of this and never finished what I set out to complete? Embarrassed and worse yet, disappointed.

> I was tired of being disappointed in myself, so quitting was not going to be an option.

I refused to go back to a time where I was unhealthy and less happy as a result. It was me that got me into this position, so it was up to me to get myself out. I had all the tools I needed; I just had to keep going one step at a time. So that is what I did . . . even in a tiny French hotel room on a work trip that provided me with more than enough excuses not to follow through.

I placed my bath towel on the floor as a workout mat, pushed the bed a little bit over to the side to make more room (let's not even discuss the filth under there), grabbed two bottles of wine to use as an extra set of weights alongside my water weights, and put my game face on to get the workout done. Were hotel room workouts like these the best of my life? No. Were they as difficult as the ones I would have done with the correct weights? No. But I remembered what Ang said:

"The only bad workout you can have is one you don't start."

To that I say, "Oui, oui!"

I was beginning to feel really good about my progress. My waist was getting smaller! I was definitely stronger and I was now capable of things I thought I never would be. I was actually visiting the gym, I could plank for a decent amount of time, and the weight and number of reps I was able to complete were steadily increasing. I even started to dabble with running, despite being worried about my knees and damaged lungs from all those years smoking. Would I just end up coughing up tar? But since I was feeling stronger in my legs and lighter overall, I had the energy—and a weird de-sire—to run. Maybe it was just because I wanted to get my 10,000 steps in faster. The last time I went for a run had to have been in high school for PE. Either way, I began by alternating jogging for one minute, then walking for one minute. As the weeks went on, I increased the running time to two minutes, then three, then four, and eventually to ten minutes with a one-minute rest. And wouldn't you believe it, I kind of enjoyed it!

My weight had fluctuated up and down a little bit week to week, which was frustrat-ing, but Ang explained that weight loss is not a linear thing . . . some weeks you lose, some you don't, and some you gain (factors such as nutrition compliance, sodium, stress, and even sleep can effect this). But as long as I continued making small chang-es over time, I knew the weight would eventually come off. By this time, I had lost 14 pounds. With sheer persistence and hard work, I earned every single one of those pounds and inches lost.

It wasn't a fast weight loss, nor was it easy, but I assure you it was weight I would never have again.

Just as I was getting into a little bit of a groove with my workouts, the end of the intensify phase meant these ones were coming to an end and would become totally different with the advanced phase to come. Time to be pushed even further out of my comfort zone. But hey, bring it on!

TERRY'S TIPS

1. You can workout anywhere . . . even in a hotel room in France.

2. You don't need your equipment to complete a workout. Wine can replace weights (as long as you don't drink it!), towels can replace mats, and you can do a lunge anywhere.

3. Continue to remind yourself why you are doing this. Make a list (write it down on paper) of reasons you need to better your health and fitness. Keep this list around and take a picture of it on your phone so you can pull it up as a motivator any time you're tempted to skip a workout.

4. On that note, keep a set of photos that inspire you on your phone too. For me, that was easy, as I already had a ton of photos of my favourite daughter.

Did I mention this is really, really hard? And lunges still suck . . . big time. But remember: You don't have to be good at every single exercise, and any workout is better than no workout . . . no excuses. Ha! Listen to me. I sound like Ang!

PLANTS

EAT SIX HANDFULS OF VEGETABLES EACH DAY

5

NUTRITION

REALITY FITNESS NUTRITION AND WORKOUT TRACKER

	Week:								Week:							
	Weight:								Weight:							
Phase	Mon	Tue	Wed	Thu	Fri	Sat	Sun	Mon	Tue	Wed	Thu	Fri	Sat	Sun	80%?
N1: 3L Water															
N2: Breakfast															
N3: Eat 3-4 hrs															
N4: Portions															
N5: Veggies															
Workouts															
10,000 steps															
Celly Countdown	5	4	3	2	1			5	4	3	2	1			
Notes:															

Newsflash: Vegetables are extremely high in essential nutrients that aid in overall health. Eating vegetables can lower your risk of cancer and help keep your digestive system on track. Eating more veggies can even help to lower your grocery bill, especially if you shop with the seasons. These are vegetable facts that we all understand; no surprise there. But this phase isn't about delving into the benefits of more vitamins or about padding your wallet. When it comes to weight loss, the purpose of veggies is really quite simple.

By volume: # calories in veggies < # calories in other foods

What makes people feel full when they eat is mostly the amount of food they consume, not the number of calories. Matching volume to calories means that while 300 calories of spinach would fill ten plates, 300 calories of pizza would fill not even one. You might be able to pound back a full pizza on your own, but what are the chances you'd be able to manage ten plates of spinach?

GAME PLAN

Eat six servings of vegetables every day.
1 serving = 1 handful or half a cup

Technically you could eat all six servings of vegetables in one sitting to comply with this phase. However, if you're keeping up with habits from previous phases, you're more likely to integrate vegetables into your meals and snacks based on your current eating schedule. For example, you could add two servings of vegetables to each meal, or you could add one vegetable serving to your breakfast and lunch, two to dinner, and then eat vegetables as part of your snacks throughout the day.

This is where you are free to ignore portions, should you so choose. If you like to eat large quantities of food, vegetables are your go-to eats.

It is not the vegetables themselves that aid in weight loss—they do not contain any sort of secret fat-burning mineral. By eating high fibre, high water content vegetables, you will feel full and less inclined to eat as much of the other high calorie foods. In this way, the addition of vegetables offsets, or in some cases replaces, other calorie-dense foods.

Because vegetables are so low in calories (provided they are not fried or doused in sauces or oils), if you wanted to incorporate more than six handfuls into your day, it would not hinder your weight loss like other higher calorie foods would. Salads, for instance, can be as large as you want when it comes to the lettuce component—the more the merrier, and the more nutrients and fibre you are going to get. Note that the more calorie dense dressings and goodies on the salad will eventually be regulated in future phases. How vegetables are prepared makes no difference to this phase (unless they are fried).

For all intents and purposes, once a vegetable is fried, it is no longer a vegetable.

Canned and frozen vegetables can be great ways to integrate more veggies into your diet, just check the label to make sure they don't have any added sugar, salt, or creams which would increase their calorie counts significantly. Cooking them several different ways helps increase variety in your meals and that will help keep you from drifting astray due to boredom. Raw, steamed, grilled, roasted, puréed into soup, added to sauces, smoothies or salsas—there's a multitude of things you can do with vegetables.

STARCHY VS. NON-STARCHY VEGETABLES

Now before you go adding a garlic-mashed potato to your dinner every night, it's important to identify the vegetables that are a hindrance to your weight loss goals. Vegetables can be separated into two categories: starchy and non-starchy. All vegetables contain fibre and nutrients that are excellent for your health, and both types are important to incorporate into a balanced and nutritious diet. But starchy vegetables are about three times higher in calories than non-starchy vegetables. Therefore, for optimal fat loss, sticking to mainly non-starchy vegetables will give you the extra edge.

> While you are free to eat as many vegetables as you please, for now, starchy vegetables do not count toward your required six handfuls for this phase.

Non-starchy vegetables are typically the flowering part of the plant. Lettuce, asparagus, broccoli, cauliflower, cucumber, spinach, mushrooms, onions, peppers, and tomatoes are a few examples of non-starchy vegetables. Some of these, as well as others, have starch in them too, but in lower levels that are not detrimental to this program. Any vegetables in this category count toward your six handfuls per day.

BUT A TOMATO IS A FRUIT!

Alright, smart-asses. Yes, tomatoes are indeed a fruit. Technically the following are botanical fruits because they contain seeds or a pit: avocado, beans, peapods, corn, cucumbers, pumpkin, squash, and (yes) tomatoes. For something to be considered a botanical vegetable, it must be something where you eat the stem, leaves, buds or roots of a plant. For example, celery (stem), lettuce (leaves), cauliflower and broccoli (buds), and carrots (roots).

This is one of those areas where common sense will prevail. For the purpose of this program, "fruits" that are lower in sugar content (such as tomatoes and cucumbers) can be consumed in larger quantities without affecting your weight loss goals. Therefore, we will consider them vegetables.

COMMON VEGETABLES

Of course there are hundreds of types of vegetables available to us via supermarkets, farmers' markets, and even in our own gardens. The next page contains a list of the most commonly chosen vegetables. More non-starchy vegetable options include: alfalfa sprouts, artichokes, bamboo shoots, bean sprouts, bok choy, brussels sprouts, cabbage, celery, chicory, daikon, eggplant, fennel, greens (e.g. collard, beet greens, dandelion, mustard, kale), green beans, hearts of palm, herbs (e.g. thyme, parsley, basil), jicama, kohlrabi, leeks, okra, radishes, rhubarb, swiss chard, and turnips.

Non-starchy

½ cup = approximately 25 calories

- Lettuce (any variety)
- Asparagus
- Broccoli
- Cauliflower
- Cucumber
- Spinach
- Mushrooms
- Onions
- Peppers (any variety)
- Tomatoes
- Carrots

Starchy

½ cup = approximately 80 calories

- Corn
- Parsnips
- Yams
- Pumpkin
- Peas
- Potatoes (any variety)
- Sweet potatoes
- Squash (any variety)
- Plantain

IDEAS FOR ADDING VEGGIES TO YOUR MENU

Vegetables are not often a favourite food, but you can learn to enjoy them (especially when you are paying attention to how they make you feel). No fancy recipes required! Sometimes all it takes is a few ideas to get the wheels turning, so here are some cooking ideas that enable you to incorporate vegetables into your diet in a way that you can enjoy while also being beneficial to your weight loss goals.

EASY

Grilled veggies: Just add just a hint of olive oil with a dash of S&P, and roast on the BBQ. Easy and tasty! Eggplant, bell peppers, asparagus, and broccoli are all great BBQ veggie options. To kick it up a notch (and to impress your buddies), you can arrange them onto skewers for vegetable kabobs.

Veggie discs: Slice a zucchini or cucumber into thin rounds, then top them with hummus or dip as you would with a regular (higher calorie) cracker.

Vegetable chili: Add extra vegetables into your regular chili recipe. You'll increase the volume of food (leftovers!) and the fibre in your meal. Celery, carrots, tomatoes, and mushrooms are great additions.

Veggie mash: instead of higher calorie potatoes, mash up cauliflower for a high-fibre, nutrient dense version. Even better, blend several types of veggies together to kick it up a notch.

QUICK VEGGIE MASH
1 cup of cauliflower, 1 cup of potato, 1 clove of garlic, 2 tbsp of yogurt.
Mash together and add a few scallions for presentation and taste.

INTERMEDIATE

Puréed soups: Soups take a bit of time but not a ton of effort to create, and they freeze well too.

BASIC PUREED VEGETABLE SOUP
Sauté olive oil, ½ cup of onions, a little garlic, and ½ cup of celery in a large pot. Add 5 cups of any other vegetables you like. Broccoli, cauliflower, carrots, zucchini, or any mixture of these make for a tasty and healthy soup. Whatever your choices, add enough broth to cover the vegetables and let simmer for about 20 minutes, then use an immersion blender to purée everything together. Add salt and pepper to taste.

Salsas: Dice ¼ cup onion, ½ tomato, ½ cup bell pepper. Add chopped cilantro, lime juice, and some salt and pepper. Mix together.

ADVANCED

Vegetable pasta: Invest in a veggie spiralizer or use a vegetable peeler to make long slivers of carrot and zucchini. Use as "noodles" on their own or blend with regular noodles before topping with a tomato-based sauce.

Stuffed vegetables: rather than dipping your vegetables into a sauce or dip, stuff veggies like mushrooms with hummus or guacamole. These types of snacks make great appetizers for parties.

Zucchini pizza: Rather than using a dough crust, use a half-inch length-wise slice of zucchini and place your toppings and cheese on top. This reduces the size of your pizza but also incorporates more vegetables, and it still tastes great!

DRINKING YOUR VEGGIES

Vegetable juice can be a great way to get in lots of veggies quickly, but store bought juice can be detrimental to your weight loss and health goals because of the amount of added sugar and sodium. Even without a juicer, you can make your own vegetable juice at home to increase your vegetable intake.

Making your own vegetable juice can be a lot of work, but you can also drink your veggies by adding them to your smoothies thereby amping up the nutrition and helping you meet your daily vegetable intake goal. If you already have a smoothie recipe you love, try adding in a handful of spinach. The smoothie will turn green, but the taste won't change much and the nutrition content and fibre content goes up exponentially.

MORE GREAT RECIPES

VEGETABLE JUICE WITH A LITTLE KICK

Ingredients

4 cups tomato, diced
½ cup carrot, diced
Small sliver of beet (mostly for colour)
1 tbsp Worcestershire sauce
½ tsp sea salt
¼ tsp cracked pepper
1 cup water, divided
¼ cup spinach
1 tbsp fresh parsley, chopped

Directions

1. Combine the tomatoes, carrots, beet sliver, Worcestershire sauce, salt, pepper, and ½ cup of the water in a small saucepan. Bring to a boil and then reduce the heat. Let simmer, covered, for 20 minutes.

2. Add the spinach and parsley and simmer for another five minutes, keeping the pan covered. Remove from heat and let cool for ten minutes.

3. Pour in blender, add remaining ½ cup of water, and purée until smooth—about two minutes. Strain through a fine-mesh sieve and serve chilled.

COCONUT BLUEBERRY SPINACH SMOOTHIE

Ingredients

⅓ cup frozen blueberries

⅔ cup baby spinach

½ cup unsweetened coconut milk

¼ cup plain Greek yogurt

1 tsp chia or hemp seeds

1 tsp maple syrup

Directions

Put all the ingredients into a blender and hit go!

EASY VEGETABLE SAUCE

Ingredients

2 tbsp olive oil

2 small onions, peeled and chopped

1 small leek, chopped

2 celery sticks, trimmed and chopped

2 red peppers, chopped

2 zucchinis, grated

2 carrots, grated

1 large pinch dried oregano

2 bay leaves

4 19-oz cans of diced tomatoes

1 small butternut squash, peeled, seeds removed, and grated

2 cups of water

1 pinch of sea salt

freshly ground black pepper to taste

This sauce is great to serve over a chicken breast or over a side of vegetables. It is also excellent in a lasagna recipe (as is or with added ground chicken or turkey). You can even make this one in bulk and freeze for future use!

Directions

1. Heat a large saucepan (big enough to hold all the ingredients) over medium heat.

2. Pour in 2 tbsp of olive oil then add the onions, leek, celery, peppers, zucchinis, carrots, and herbs. Cook everything together for about 20 minutes with the lid on, until all the vegetables are nice and soft.

3. Add the tomatoes, squash, water, salt, and pepper to the vegetables. Bring to a boil and simmer gently for about 30 minutes until the squash is soft.

4. Fish out the bay leaves and allow the sauce to cool slightly before blending until smooth. Taste and season with a little more salt and pepper if needed.

ASPARAGUS GUACAMOLE

Ingredients

½ pound asparagus, trimmed

1 avocado, pitted and peeled

1 Serrano pepper (seeds and membranes removed for less heat)

Juice of ½ lime

2 garlic cloves, minced

¼ cup red onion, diced or minced

¼ cup cilantro, minced

1 tomato, chopped

Directions

1. Place asparagus stalks in a steamer over 1 inch of boiling water; cover and wait until they're bright green and tender, 3-5 minutes. Remove from steamer. When cool, cut into ½ inch pieces.

2. Purée asparagus in a food processor or blender. Add avocado, Serrano pepper, lime juice, and garlic. Pulse until guacamole is desired texture.

3. Stir in red onion, cilantro, and tomato. Season with salt and pepper.

It did not come as a surprise when Ang said I was going to be adding more vegetables into my daily diet. I knew the day would come, but I was flabbergasted when she said I had to (somehow) add six handfuls of vegetables to this process. Six servings sounded like a lot. Turns out I was right.

I know vegetables are healthy, but I didn't like to eat them and never really took notice when I hadn't had any in a while. Sometimes a long while, unless the pickle on a burger counts. It took me about one day to realize how few vegetables I was actually eating prior to this phase. I certainly wasn't asking for them as one of my side options at a restaurant (I usually opted for the loaded potato, fries, pasta, or rice). And yet, if you were to ask me then if I was eating vegetables, I would have probably said yes.

> It is almost as if because it requires such an effort to choose and eat vegetables, you really overplay the memories of the times you do eat them to make it feel like a real accomplishment.

My plan at the beginning of this challenge was to simply eat all six handfuls of veggies at once to get it over with. Similar to the exercise, if I could just get it all done as soon as possible, then I didn't have the burden hanging over me all day. I don't recommend this approach, unless you enjoy sitting in front of a mound of veggies and gnawing away at them for about an hour. My stomach didn't care for it much either. And Diane, well she will definitely tell you it was not a good idea, as she had to live with me after I ate all that roughage! No need for details, I'm sure you get the idea. After only one successful attempt to eat all six handfuls of veggies in one sitting, I changed my strategy to a more balanced approach—two handfuls at each meal. I needed to spread the servings out throughout the day so that I didn't feel like exploding. Plus, I was having trouble adding in any other foods when I ate that many veggies at one time.

I started with breakfast by adding some spinach into my morning smoothie. My blue smoothies were now green smoothies and looked really gross, but I swear that when you mix it up you cannot taste it! Boom. Two handfuls of veggies already in for the day every morning.

Next I integrated some of what Ang called "veggie satchels" into my snacks or as part of my lunch. These were raw veggies cut up and portioned into bags or containers. I made these well in advance so I didn't get put off at the idea of having to prepare them (it can take a lot of time in the middle of the day!). With the satchels ready to go, I didn't have to think about anything other than chewing.

Finally at supper, I would have two more handfuls of either steamed or roasted vegetables. Grilled asparagus is a nice treat in season (did I just call a vegetable a treat?!). Grilled mushrooms, stuffed bell peppers or a salad topped with blue cheese are some of my other favourites. Sometimes salad got boring, so Ang suggested some "fancy" options for vegetables in the form of stir-fries, puréed soups, or even some salads that had no lettuce. These were things I didn't really have time for (maybe later when I'm fully retired)!

During this particular phase I was travelling a lot for work, and let me tell you, it was not easy to make vegetables a part of my regular day.

I had to plan to make it happen.

For domestic travel I would pack a veggie satchel for everyday I was away, and I always made sure in advance that my hotels had a mini-fridge to keep them fresh. If I was travelling overseas, I picked up pre-cut veggie trays and little baggies at a supermarket and made all my satchels in the hotel room prior to my first day of meetings. I did encounter a couple of trips where I literally did not have time to stop at a supermarket, so I asked the hotel restaurant to pack me a salad for every day I was in town and kept them in my mini fridge so I was prepared. (I know. I'm hard-core now!)

Prior to this phase, I could not tell you the last time I had a salad or even a tomato or cucumber on my plate. But now, vegetables are the first thing I think of when I go to make my meal. It seems hard at first, but after sitting down to make a veggie plan, things begin to look a little less daunting.

I'm not sure if the added veggies were working at the time or not, but when I got home one particular evening during this phase (after two weeks of travelling) I stepped on the scale and nearly lost my mind. I was up to a 21-pound loss now! I did not miss a single day of veggies, but I am sure it was a combination of everything—not just the vegetables, but the regular eating and portioning too. The program was working, and I was so thrilled!

Bottom line: vegetables make you feel full, and if you feel full, you eat less of the other crap.

I did not remember ever feeling unsatisfied or like I was missing out on something. Plus, I felt more energetic, lighter, and less foggy. I hope you'll feel the same once you get this phase under way.

> I can't say that I now love vegetables or ever have a crazy craving for a chunk of broccoli, but I can say that as long as I plan which vegetables I am going to incorporate into each meal, I am guaranteed to get them in. Having a plan is key.

If I'm not organized with a plan and have not pre-cut them or set them aside for a certain meal, it does not happen. And I would say that is true to this day (over five years later), not just in the first few weeks of trying this out. Be prepared! Of all the habits, this is one of the easiest to let slide. It takes effort to be organized, and a real awareness of what you are doing to have consistent success with this one. Oh man, I sound like Ang. Time to crack a celly beer!

TERRY'S TIPS

1. Prepare your vegetables as soon as you're home from the store. It takes no more than 20 minutes; I've timed it. Chop them and portion them into satchels or package them for your own salad bar throughout the week. If you wait a few hours after you get home, you are much less likely to wash them and cut them up.

2. Add treats into your salads! Salads don't have to be only vegetables. Provided you don't add too much (which can counter your weight loss progress), adding some small bits of cheese, meat, nuts, or fresh herbs such as basil, mint, or tarragon can pack salads with a ton of flavour and help kill salad boredom.

3. Always choose the veggie side. Even if they aren't on the menu, most restaurants can accommodate a request for veggies along side the main instead of fries.

4. Fresh salsa. This became one of my favourites. It was easy to eat on its own (with a few chips . . . but I did not say that), or I would put it on top of a chicken breast or grilled fish for an easy meal.

5. Two handfuls of veggies is half your plate if you're eating off the smaller one. Thinking of it this way makes for easy tracking.

TERRY'S VEGGIE SATCHELS

Ingredients

1 bunch of celery

6 large carrots

2 bell peppers (any colour)

2 bunches of radishes

These veggies make approximately six large satchels for the week. If my wife wanted some for the week too, I doubled the formula. These particular veggies tend to last all week long versus veggies such as cucumbers or tomatoes that are softer and tend to go gooey in a few days.

PLANNING CELLIES

*GRADUALLY DECREASING, BUT
DEFINITELY **NOT** ELIMINATING TREATS*

Part Two

CELLIES

REALITY FITNESS NUTRITION AND WORKOUT TRACKER

	Week:								Week:							
	Weight:								Weight:							
	Mon	Tue	Wed	Thu	Fri	Sat	Sun		Mon	Tue	Wed	Thu	Fri	Sat	Sun	80%?
Phase																
N1: 3L Water																
N2: Breakfast																
N3: Eat 3-4 hrs																
N4: Portions																
N5: Veggies																
10,000 steps																
Workouts																
Celly Countdown		3	2	1					3	2	1					

Notes:

Notice how easy it is to just grab a little candy off someone's desk, or to have just one more beer with the boys before you head out? These choices are not calorie-free! Just because it wasn't on a plate does not mean you didn't eat it.

GAME PLAN

Limit your cellies to three or less a week.

Now that you are aware of what a celly is, and you have had practice keeping track of five or less in a week, it is time to up the ante. Just to reinforce: we will not get to a point in the program where all indulgences are taken out of your diet. This is not a realistic goal, and it would likely be very difficult to sustain long term . . . and quite frankly just not much fun.

Remember: It's not necessarily the types of foods or drinks themselves that make us fat, it's the quantity in which we have them.

EXTRA SCOOPS OF HEALTHY FOOD COUNTS

It's not only treats and alcohol that can throw you off your program game. A piece of pie for dessert can be equally as derailing as an extra pork chop or roll at dinnertime.

Now that you are well-versed in portioning, cellies now mean extra helpings of healthy foods too.

So, if you're adding an extra scoop of rice to your plate, that's a celly. Indulging in an extra-large portion of steak? That's also a celly. Lucky for you, though, extra non-starchy vegetables on your plate (provided they are not smothered in butter and salt) don't count as a celly. You can still eat as many of those as you want!

PLAN YOUR WEEK IN ADVANCE

You have probably already discovered that in order to adhere to your weekly celly limits, you have to plan your day in advance, if not your entire week, to not risk over-doing it. Considering the week that lies ahead of you, and planning for your cellies accordingly, can go a long way in terms of your success with this program. If you know there's a party on Friday night and a brunch on Sunday morning, you can plan to save your cellies for these days and avoid the temptation of grabbing a random handful of jelly beans at the office on Wednesday or of saying yes to the stale cookies offered to you on a plane.

Plan your cellies around holidays or special occasions first. If you don't have any of these during the week, plan your indulgences around foods or restaurants you truly love.

> Don't waste your cellies on random things that aren't amazing to you or that just happen along your day. Make your cellies worth it, and savour every bite!

I'm the kind of guy that always does better with a plan to keep me on track. When it came to my meals, I was very disciplined each week and was confident I was eating reasonable sized portions by the end of phase four. With all of my meals on track, I looked at my calendar at the start of each week to strategically plan where I would add in my cellies. A pattern quickly emerged. I was certainly not going to give up a glass of wine on Friday nights with Diane—that was our date night! Saturday I usually planned a beer after golf. And Sunday was ice cream or a few chicken wings while watching Tiger Woods bat it around on TV. Believe it or not, sometimes days came about where I didn't feel like having my planned celly, so I skipped it or saved it for another day. This didn't happen all that often, but sometimes I surprised myself.

> One thing I noticed was how I began to appreciate my cellies so much more than I used to. Now they were special, and it even made the moments and people I shared them with special.

I know, I know. Now I'm getting sappy! Anyway, I guess that is what cellies are supposed to be—a treat and a celebration. If you have them any time you want, or all the time, they become less special and your appreciation for them decreases.

But it's scary how easily you can slip back into your old ways! Another scoop of something delicious, then an extra snack here, and a grab of something there almost led me down a path where I was risking going back to where I started. Over the holidays I found I was giving myself permission to indulge because that is what I used to do. My weight loss stalled—the efforts with all my meal planning, meal preparation, and suffering exercise were not having their benefits because of the handfuls of candies, chocolates, and nuts I was eating out of the snowflake dishes sitting decoratively and tempting me on our coffee table. Gaining weight back could not be an option for me, I decided, so that left me with two choices:

1. Continue to work really hard at the planning, prep, and exercise while still eating all my favourite treats and extras, and be okay with not losing weight for a few weeks.

2. Choose to stick with my plan, focus on my goal, and push on!

I know that for the purpose of this book it would probably sound so good if I told you I chose option 2 and felt so proud afterward and it was so worth it and it will be for you too. But seriously? Shit, I'm only human! I did all the habits and exercises to a T with the exception of the cellies. I just ate and drank too many . . . for about two weeks straight! I did not gain any weight, though. Was I healthier? No. Was I happy about it? No. But I did continue following the program and this made me feel good since I wanted to keep those changes ingrained. And by doing this I did not feel like I had to "start over" by the time the holidays were over. I just went back to limiting my cellies again and the weight started to come down about two weeks later. I guess you could say I had about one month of a plateau with the weight loss because of my holiday indulgences, but maintaining the rest of the program in the meantime saved my ass so I could pick right back up and move on!

TERRY'S TIPS

1. I sure give a lot of tips in this book. How's this for a tip: just listen to what Ang says! She hasn't steered you wrong yet.

MUSCLE FUEL

INCORPORATE PROTEIN INTO
EVERY MEAL AND SNACK

6

NUTRITION

REALITY FITNESS NUTRITION AND WORKOUT TRACKER

	Week:							Week:						
	Weight:							Weight:						
Phase	Mon	Tue	Wed	Thu	Fri	Sat	Sun	Mon	Tue	Wed	Thu	Fri	Sat	Sun
N1: 3L Water														80%?
N2: Breakfast														
N3: Eat 3-4 hrs														
N4: Portions														
N5: Veggies														
N6: Protein														
10,000 steps														
Workouts														
Celly Countdown		3	2	1					3	2	1			

Comments:

Your body's muscle is responsible for burning calories. The more muscle you have on your body, the more calories your body burns even when you're at rest or sleeping. Protein is the building block for developing and maintaining lean muscle mass and is therefore a crucial element to successful weight loss.

GAME PLAN

Eat protein as a part of every meal and snack.

Further to your muscles being responsible for burning calories, it takes more energy for your body to process protein foods such as chicken, fish, and nuts than it does to process carbohydrate foods like bread, rice, and pasta. For example, it takes about five to ten calories for your body to process a slice of bread of about 100 calories. In comparison, if you eat 100 calories of meat, the energy required to process it is about 20-30 calories. This is nearly three times the energy required than that for processing carbohydrate foods.

Protein has a slew of other benefits to weight loss, as well. The addition of protein foods improves the function of the hormone leptin, which signals the brain to let it know you are full, thereby reducing hunger and overeating. This is one reason why you feel fuller for longer after you eat a turkey breast (protein food) versus a cup of pasta (carbohydrate food).

Protein is also helpful in reducing fat storage by instructing the hormone insulin to work efficiently in the muscle. This helps muscles maintain their mass, but also helps them use glucose (sugar) as fuel (versus storing it as fat) to aid in healthy insulin function.

Protein also has a thermic effect. The thermic effect of food refers to the heat generated from increased energy output during the digestion period. The heat generated by your body can be extrapolated and thought of as a little mini-workout. It spikes your metabolism ever so slightly that you are actually burning more calories after you eat it versus when you eat other foods, since carbohydrates and fats have a much lower thermic effect than protein. Therefore, eating two eggs in the morning (protein food) instead of two slices of toast (carbohydrate food) can boost weight loss because the protein wakes up your liver (the metabolic powerhouse of your body) and provides it with something substantial to process.

Carbohydrates and fats are much easier for the liver to process where as protein requires more effort. Much like your workouts, the more effort you have to put in, the harder it is, but the more calories you burn.

Please do not take this phase as a reason to eat an entire chicken for dinner!

Remember your portion sizes from phase four; you are to incorporate protein into your meals and snacks within the portions set out for you then. Integrating protein into your phase four portions looks like a palm-size amount at every meal and a handful at every snack.

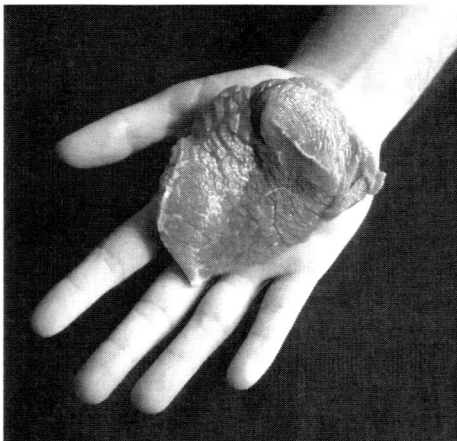

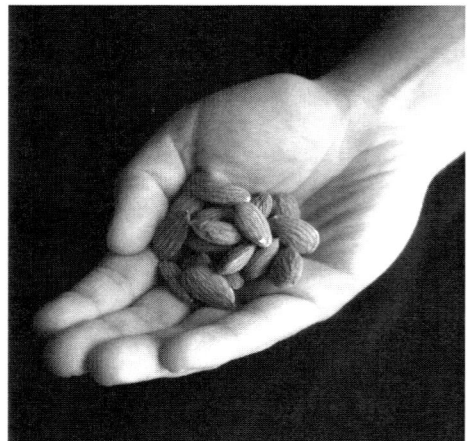

The amount of protein should fit easily in the cup of your hand (not overflowing).

Many types of foods have protein in them, but certain foods provide more protein than others. Your meals should incorporate 30 grams of protein (20 grams for women). With your limited portion sizes, animal protein such as meat, fish, and eggs are the best options for meals. For snacks, try nuts, seeds, edamame, tofu, or dairy products like yogurt or cheese. Foods such as beans, lentils, and grains high in protein (think faro or quinoa) can be included as well, but know that with these you will not consume nearly as much protein as you would with meat products (assuming you stay within the appropriate portion size) and therefore will not receive the same benefits of the protein, including the increased muscle mass and caloric burn.

PROTEIN POWDERS

If you are using protein powders, again 30 grams is sufficient (20 grams for women). Whey protein is ideal, though casein protein powder and egg white protein powder are also acceptable, as are hemp, pea, beef, and veggie protein powders for those who are vegetarian or vegan. Protein powders can be purchased at most health and vitamin stores, supermarkets, and often at fitness stores.

> Be careful. Just because these powders can be purchased at "health" stores does not mean they are always "healthy."

Be sure to check the labels and select a powder that has minimal ingredients listed. The fewer the ingredients, the more natural the product is. If it takes you more than ten seconds to read the label, put the product down and look for another one.

> Ideally you will chew your meals versus drinking them.

When adding protein powders into your nutrition repertoire, opt to add in just one protein powder snack or meal a day. Believe it or not, research has shown that chewing your food provides more satisfaction than drinking it. If you are more satisfied, the less likely you are to stray. Powders are indeed an excellent source of protein and are really helpful when in a hurry, but ideally you'll be getting in a variety of protein types, including those in non-liquid form. Learning to plan and prepare regular meals takes practice but is much more sustainable in the long run versus drinking all of your meals.

ADDING VARIETY

There is no expectation that you limit yourself to a bland chicken breast everyday. With a little effort, you can add a ton of variety to your meals.

> Food, like life, is not meant to be boring.

It's amazing how a different cooking technique can completely change the flavour of food. You can grill, poach, bake, roast, broil or smoke, among many other ways. Using spices and techniques from other cultures can also greatly affect the taste and texture of your protein sources. Think about how the flavour of salmon is altered when you bake it with salt, add some dill, or drizzle it with teriyaki sauce. Here are some recipes to help with adding variety to your meals.

MEXICAN CHICKEN BURRITOS WITH BLACK BEANS

Ingredients
1 15-oz can black beans, drained and rinsed
1 cup shredded rotisserie chicken breast
½ cup shredded cheddar cheese
½ tsp cumin
½ tsp pepper
½ tsp kosher salt
8 corn tortillas
non-stick cooking spray

Directions
1. Preheat oven to 375°F and spray a large cookie sheet generously with non-stick cooking spray. Coat it well enough to see a thin layer of oil.

2. In a medium mixing bowl, combine black beans, chicken, cheese, and spices. Divide mixture evenly among tortillas. Roll tortillas around filling and hold closed with toothpicks.

3. Place on prepared cookie sheet. Spray tops of burritos generously with non-stick cooking spray.

4. Bake for 6 minutes, then turn burritos over and bake for another 6-8 minutes, until golden. Remove toothpicks and serve.

DILL TURKEY BURGERS

Ingredients

1 lb ground turkey
¼ cup finely chopped dill pickles
2 tsp fresh dill
1 tbsp lemon pepper
¾ cup whole grain bread crumbs
1 egg
whole grain hamburger buns

Directions

1. Mix all of the ingredients together and form into 4 patties about ½ inch thick.

2. Cook on the BBQ until cooked all the way through.

3. Serve with your condiments of choice.

MOROCCAN-SPICED WHITE FISH

Ingredients

2 tbsp extra-virgin olive oil
½ cup shallots or onion, thinly sliced
2 garlic cloves, minced
¾ tsp ground cumin
½ tsp cinnamon
1 15-oz can diced tomatoes
Juice and grated zest of 1 medium lemon
4 6-oz pieces of white fish (e.g. halibut, orange roughy, or hake; frozen is fine)
¼ tsp salt
¼ tsp freshly ground pepper
¼ cup cilantro or flat leaf parsley, whole or roughly chopped

Directions

1. Heat oil in a 12-inch heavy skillet over medium heat. Add the shallots and cook until slightly softened, about 2-3 minutes. Add the garlic, cumin, and cinnamon, stir for 1 minute longer.

2. Stir in tomatoes, lemon juice, zest, salt, and pepper. Simmer uncovered, stirring occasionally, until thickened, about 10 minutes.

3. Pat fish dry and season both sides with salt and pepper. Add fish to skillet. Cover and simmer until fish is just cooked through, 7-10 minutes. Serve with hot cooked couscous or rice and sprinkle with cilantro or parsley.

THAI STYLE CHICKEN

Ingredients

⅓ cup fresh basil

⅓ cup fresh mint

⅓ cup cilantro

3 tbsp fresh ginger, peeled and chopped

4 garlic cloves, peeled

1 ½ tbsp soy sauce

1 ½ tbsp fish sauce

1 ½ tbsp olive oil

1 ½ tbsp honey

1 Serrano chilli, stemmed and chopped

6 skinless boneless chicken breast halves (about 2 ½ lbs total)

Directions

1. Combine first 10 ingredients in a food processor. Process until well blended, scraping down sides of bowl occasionally.

2. Arrange chicken in a medium-sized glass dish. Spoon herb mixture over chicken, covering completely. Cover dish and chill at least 2 hours, turning chicken occasionally. (Can be made a day ahead. Keep chilled.)

3. When ready to cook, prepare BBQ and set to medium-high heat. Grill the chicken until cooked through, about 5 minutes per side.

4. Cut chicken crosswise into thin slices. Transfer to plates and serve with brown rice and a selection of grilled vegetables.

WEEKLY MEAL PLANS

Establishing a consistent weekly protein meal plan can help simplify the decisions on what to eat, recipes to search for, or even what restaurant to go to. Here is a sample weekly meal plan.

WEEKLY PROTEIN MEAL IDEAS

Monday:	Chicken Night	Roasted chicken or a chicken breast
Tuesday:	Beef Night	A nice lean cut of steak
Wednesday:	Fish Night	Salmon or tilapia
Thursday:	Meatless Night	Beans/lentils/vegetarian option
Friday:	Turkey Night	Turkey burgers
Saturday:	Seafood Night	Scallops or shrimp
Sunday:	Something Different Night	Bison, elk, or pork

Oh boy, another step to add to my already altered eating habits. It was getting more challenging week after week to make these small changes, but I was seeing the number on the scale go down and, to my surprise, even some definition developing in my arms, shoulders, and chest, so that kept me going. This next phase was all about adding protein to my meals and snacks. My first question for Ang was: "What the hell is protein?" I had heard the word a bunch of times before on TV, but I never really understood what it actually was or how to eat it. This was something that had always bugged me about nutrition—people in-the-know seemed to use lingo that the rest of us didn't understand. I just took it for jargon that allowed others to sound smarter than they actually were, so I was always skeptical of their information. Now that my favourite daughter was using the P word with me, I guess I was gonna have to change my opinion.

> As soon as Ang explained what protein actually was, and once I understood that it would help me build muscle and lose weight, I wanted to know more.

I had no idea that protein is a component of many foods—from meat to cheese to nuts—that helps build muscle. I thought protein was a solitary ingredient you could buy at the market in the same way you'd buy milk. Seriously, years of hearing the word protein and never really understanding what it meant. Now I do! Ang listed off foods that were high in protein and gave me suggestions on how to cook them for my meals and incorporate them into my snacks. I felt confident that I'd easily be able to make protein a part of my lifestyle.

It all seemed pretty easy at first. I was already doing okay with breakfast because I had eggs or a smoothie every morning. I never associated my smoothies with protein. (That word comes up all the time now and drives me crazy!) Now I add protein sources like yogurt or whey powder. For lunches and dinners I made sure to have some sort of meat or fish to get the protein serving in there. It was a rare occasion for me not to have meat at a meal anyway, so this wasn't hard. Keeping to the correct portion, of course, remained a challenge!

If I was travelling I kept my protein selections as local as possible. This was my way of keeping it interesting and eating fresh food. Near the coast I typically opted for the seafood—shrimp, crab, lobster, scallops. If I was landlocked, I went with land-dwellers like chicken, turkey, or beef.

It was the snacks that were tricky. I really did not want to be eating a chicken breast at 10:00 am, or too much meat all day, for that matter. My solutions became hard boiled eggs, nuts, and seeds. Thank goodness for these! They were easy to portion, portable, and quick to eat when I was on the go. And you can buy nuts and seeds almost anywhere!

> There is no excuse. Every airport in North America sells some sort of satchel of nuts. You just have to have the discipline to choose the nuts and not the chocolate bar next to them.

I even discovered little packets of to-go Justin's Natural Almond Butter in a magazine store in Houston. Perfect for a little protein burst! The day I discovered them I had to text Ang a photo, I was so pumped! (Seriously? Did I just say that?) Another one of my favourite tricks when travelling was to pack individual baggies of protein powder that I could easily add into an instant oatmeal from a coffee shop. Was this a perfect meal? No. But at least it was a little extra protein, and the serving size was typically within reason.

While the protein phase of this program seemed simple on its own, the whole food planning aspect at this stage of the program in general, between eating often and portioning and eating veggies and selecting protein, was becoming a monumental change that was getting hard to keep up. It felt like it took more time to plan my food than it did to eat it! At first I was worried I would not be able to succeed because the effort to plan seemed so taxing. I had enough lists in my life! Correcting my mindset would be critical to my continued determination.

> I focused on the positive alterations instead of the difficulty of the changes and reminded myself of why this was important to endure.

My health (or lack thereof) before starting the program was distracting me from living my life, and I was ready—I needed—for that not to be the case anymore. I was finished with feeling ashamed of my fitness level, of my waistline, and I wanted to rid myself of the guilt associated with not following through on what I had always said I would do. Now or never, and I was seeing the results. My waistline was shrinking slowly, yes, but regardless of the numbers I was waking up with more energy every day, and I'll be damned if I can't say that I was just generally a happier guy. Finally, I had committed to a single program, I was executing it to the best of my ability every day, and it was working. The effort was challenging, but the results felt so good! Why would I quit now? Ang was so proud, I couldn't let her down. I had to keep going.

> So eating protein at every meal and snack takes a bit of planning, but it is worth it.

This phase helped me stay full and also helped me lose some weight. I'm sure it was the combination of the other phases that started bringing on bigger changes, but they really became noticeable throughout this phase. The only bad thing? By the end of this phase I realized that I'm now one of those guys that says *protein* all the time. I can't believe it. What has happened to me?!

TERRY'S TIPS

1. Portion out your nuts, cheese, yogurt, and hard-boiled eggs ahead of time, because it is really easy to overeat these foods—they are just so tasty!

2. Cook a few turkey breasts or lean steaks on the weekend and add them to salads throughout the week. The less cooking/planning during the workweek, the better!

3. Make use of your BBQ. Consider it your new best friend! It is such an easy way to cook protein foods. It seems to taste so much better, and it's also an easier (and less time consuming) clean up.

4. Establish a consistent weekly protein meal-plan. For example, every Monday is chicken night, every Wednesday is beef, Fridays is seafood, etc. It's easier for making decisions on what to eat, recipes to search for, or even what restaurant to go to in an evening, and it limits the amount of planning you have to do each week too

EAT FAT
TO LOSE FAT

EAT A SERVING OF FAT IN EVERY MEAL AND SNACK

NUTRITION

REALITY FITNESS NUTRITION AND WORKOUT TRACKER

	Week:								Week:							
	Weight:								Weight:							
Phase	Mon	Tue	Wed	Thu	Fri	Sat	Sun	Mon	Tue	Wed	Thu	Fri	Sat	Sun	80%?
N1: 3L Water															
N2: Breakfast															
N3: Eat 3-4 hrs															
N4: Portions															
N5: Veggies															
N6: Protein															
N7: Fat															
10,000 steps															
Workouts															
Celly Countdown		3	2	1					3	2	1				

Notes:

For many reasons, healthy fats actually aid in fat loss. They are high in calories and stay in your stomach longer, contributing to a more satisfied feeling that can result in less overeating. Healthy fats also boost your liver's role in releasing the fat you don't want. Without healthy fats in the diet, the liver doesn't work properly and your body stores unwanted fat instead. Therefore, incorporating a bit of healthy fat into your nutrition plan is very important for weight loss and overall health. There are many other benefits too, from better heart health to enabling your body to better absorb nutrients like Vitamins A, D, E, and K. Not to mention the benefits fat has on your joint health to support your workouts.

GAME PLAN

Incorporate one serving—no more, no less—of healthy fat to every meal and snack you eat. When in doubt, one tablespoon is a serving size, or about the size of the tip of your thumb, from the knuckle up.

Of course too much healthy fat, being as high in calories as it is (nine calories in a single gram, or more than double the calories of a single gram of carbohydrate or protein), can lead to weight gain if eaten in too large of quantities. Again, since weight loss is primarily about calories in versus calories out, it is important not to overeat even healthy fats—which can be hard because they taste so great! The following section outlines your healthy fat choices.

FAT OPTIONS AND PORTIONS

For the purposes of this program, the naturally occurring fats in meat do not count toward your healthy fat consumption.

BEST FATS
- 1 tbsp of healthy oil (see section on oils for more information)
- 1 egg (yolk)
- A small handful of nuts or seeds (¼ cup)
- 2 tbsp of avocado
- 1 tbsp oil-based salad dressing (e.g. Italian)

For those eating two eggs for breakfast, switch to one full egg and two egg whites to stick within the guidelines.

ACCEPTABLE FATS
- 1 tbsp of butter
- 1 tbsp of mayonnaise
- 1 tbsp of creamy salad dressing
- 1 oz of cheese

Often this phase goes unnoticed in terms of how you feel, as you're likely already getting the fat you need in your diet. If you are already eating nuts as your protein snack, for example, it will not be necessary to add more fat as you can count the fat in the nuts as your protein and your fat.

The only time it feels like a dramatic alteration is when the portion size is considered. Often the proper serving size is a lot smaller than people realize.

BEWARE OF CAMO-FAT!
Camo-fat is fat that is hidden, but still present. A salad with a tablespoon of dressing is perfect. But as soon as you add nuts or seeds and cheese, you've possibly tripled your allowed fat content.

DIFFERENT KINDS OF FAT

There are several kinds of fats, and they are not all equal. Some are healthy and contribute to weight loss and overall health, while others are detrimental to your well-being and your waistline. The three fat varieties are unsaturated fats, also known as monounsaturated and polyunsaturated fats (the healthy kind); saturated fats (the less healthy kind); and trans fats (the very unhealthy kind).

Polyunsaturated and monounsaturated fats are healthy fats that help maintain normal cholesterol levels, and have been shown to reduce the risk of heart disease. Omega 3s found in salmon and walnuts are both excellent sources of this type of fat.

Saturated fats—found in beef, butter, and dairy products such as cream, milk, and cheese—should be minimized. These fats are natural but can contribute to high cholesterol in the blood if overeaten. These types of fats found in meat products do not count as your healthy fat for this phase and do not have to be omitted, but aim to eat them less often. For example, keep red meat consumption to once or twice a week and stick to leaner choices the rest of the week. Cheese and butter, however, can be easily tracked and accounted for, so do consider these your one fat choice if it is present at any meal or snack. Sound complicated? That's okay! Use the Reality Fitness Protein/Carb/Fat Options & Portions chart (Appendix C) as your guide. Select one fat from the list at every meal and snack, opting for the "best" options as often as possible for optimal health.

Avoid trans fats altogether, as these are linked to visceral belly fat, which contributes to Type 2 Diabetes and can lead to heart disease and certain cancers. Trans fats are often found in margarines, packaged snack foods, pre-baked items, processed meats, and some brands of nut butters. If the packaging contains the words "partially hydrogenated" on the front or in the ingredient list, the product contains trans fats and you should put it back on the shelf.

VISCERAL BELLY FAT
Visceral fat is body fat that is stored within the abdominal cavity and is therefore stored around a number of important internal organs such as the liver, pancreas, and intestines. Visceral fat is sometimes referred to as 'active fat' because research has shown that this type of fat plays a distinctive and potentially dangerous role affecting how our hormones function.

COOKING WITH OIL

The oil that you use to cook with does count toward your fat intake for the day. That said, if you do not cook with it properly (i.e. if you cook a specific oil at too high a temperature), you can break down the oil into parts that are no longer useful—and potentially harmful—to your body. The breakdown releases free radicals as well as a substance called acrolein, a chemical that gives burnt foods their acrid flavour and aroma.

When cooking with monounsaturated and polyunsaturated fats, note that each fat or oil has a unique use. Some fats and oils are made for high heat cooking, while others have intense flavours that are best enjoyed drizzled directly onto food.

The temperature that is required to make oil smoke is called the smoke point. When cooking at high temperatures, choose an oil or fat with a very high smoke point. In general, the lighter the colour of the oil, the higher its smoke point. Most foods are cooked between temperatures of 350-450° Fahrenheit, so it is best to choose an oil or fat with a smoke point above 400°F.

OILS AND THEIR SMOKE POINTS

Oils that work well for oiling frying pans and cooking above 350°F:
- Almond: 420°F
- Avocado: 520°F
- Grapeseed: 392°F
- Olive (Ex. Light): 468°F
- Olive (Virgin):   420° F
- Peanut: 450°F
- Sesame: 410°F
- Sunflower: 450°F

Oils that are excellent to drizzle over salads, used in baking, or for cooking below 350°F:
- Butter: 350°F
- Coconut oil: 350°F
- Olive (Ex. Virgin): 320°F

(Use butter and coconut oil less often due to saturated fat.)

When Ang asked me to start adding fat into my meals and snacks I was shocked! In my mind, fat was what made you fat, so why on earth would I start eating more of it? My goodness! At this point I had put in all this work, and now I was going to add in something I thought I was supposed to avoid? This made no sense to me, and it made me nervous that I would stop seeing progress or—worse—gain back what I had already lost!

Turns out I was worried for nothing. Ang explained to me the differences in kinds of fat, and I realized that I was already eating some healthy fats.

> I thought just deep fried foods were fat. I didn't realize healthy foods had fat too.

For example, my boiled eggs that I ate on occasion for a snack had a portion of fat in them due to the yolk, so I did not need to add anything extra. Same for the nuts. Healthy fat: check. I didn't know it in the beginning, but finally I was in the position of having already been doing something right!

For me, I mostly needed to think about how to add fats to lunch and supper, and suddenly being aware of what they were kinda threw my mind for a loop. Sounds silly, I know, because I was already eating fats on a regular basis before this phase. But for some reason, once I knew what foods I was eating that had fat in them, those old "myths" about fat making you fat began to trickle in and make me paranoid about their consumption. Ang had to be on my case about it!

"Dad, did you get your fat in today?"

"Dad, are you eating your fat?"

"Dad. Your fat. Did you eat it?"

"Dad. Eat your fat."

It's funny how we can get hung up on certain ideas about nutrition (whether they are true or not). These barriers take time to overcome, and I eventually did.

I found it easy to track the fat for my meals. A tablespoon of oil for cooking or of dressing for salad, and I was covered. Avocados have the good fats in them too, and I have a great recipe for guacamole that I use as a sandwich spread. I'll leave it at the end of this chapter. For snacks, however, it got tricky because of the protein/fat overlap for foods that counted as both. When it came to double-duty foods, I opted for a quarter-cup of nuts. While I wanted to double my portion (I did need a fat *and* a protein, afterall), I knew this was a cheat since the nuts counted as my portion for *both* fat and protein at once.

> When I was finally eating them, I did find not overdoing healthy fats a challenge for this step. With a tiny serving size of one thumb or about one tablespoon, it is really easy to add "just a little bit more" salad dressing or to have "a few more" nuts, which added up to a lot of extra calories.

Did you know you have to run for almost thirty minutes at six miles an hour to burn off a few extra tablespoons of some salad dressings? I suppose I could use a celly for the extra dressing or integrate more of a workout to balance it out, if I wanted, but a cost/benefit analysis of drizzling an extra bit over my salad helped me come to the realization that if I was going to go that way I would rather have a beer!

> Strive for the correct portion size, save the calories, and have a beer!

TERRY'S TIPS

1. Measure out your fats. They are high in calories, so any extra you pay for! I don't know about you, but I did not want to waste any extra time in the gym for a few extra nuts. Measure out small bags of nuts or cheese ahead of time to add to a salad or eat as a snack. This reduces the chance of tossing on "just a few more." Measuring out salad dressing in little containers (even if you are not taking your meal to go) also saves you a lot of calories versus pouring from the container.

2. Choose foods that serve more than one purpose. Two birds, one bite. For example, the almonds I had at my snack were considered protein and fat . . . no need to add extra fat. Consider these foods the biggest bang for your efforts, as you only have to eat one serving to get two benefits. This is what I kept telling myself instead of feeling ripped off that I didn't get to add in more food!

This phase was not very noticeable for me. For weeks I thought I was doing something wrong because it seemed to make no real difference. I guess in the long run it had an impact because I lost the weight eventually, but during the process it felt like one more thing to think about, and often it was an afterthought. Like I said, a lot of the foods that I was already eating had healthy fats in them. I was finished the phase before I even started it!

Oh yeah, and here's that guac recipe I promised you.

TERRY'S AMPED UP SANDWICH SAUCE: GUACAMOLE

Ingredients

3 avocados, peeled, pitted, and mashed

1 lime, juiced

1 tsp salt

½ cup onion, chopped

3 tbsp fresh cilantro, chopped

2 roma (plum) tomatoes, diced

1 tsp garlic, minced

1 pinch ground cayenne pepper (optional)

Directions

1. In a medium bowl, mash together the avocados, lime juice, and salt.

2. Add onion, cilantro, tomatoes, and garlic. Mix.

3. Stir in cayenne pepper.

4. Serve immediately or, for best flavour, refrigerate at least one hour.

REALITY FITNESS
ADVANCED PHASE

FASTER, LONGER, STRONGER!

YOU'RE GOING TO FEEL A SENSATION

Advanced

FITNESS

REALITY FITNESS ASSESSMENT TRACKING FORM

	BUILDING	INTENSIFY	ADVANCED	SUSTAINABILITY		
DATE OF ASSESSMENT						
TIME OF DAY						
BODY COMPOSITION						
Weight						
Neck						
Shoulders						
Chest						
Waist						
Hips						
Right Arm						
Right Leg						
CARDIOVASCULAR FITNESS						
1.5 mile run time						
OR						
1.0 mile walk time						
MUSCULAR ENDURANCE						
Squats (# in 1 minute)						
Pushups Off Toes (max #)						
OR						
Pushups Off Knees (max #)						
Plank off Elbows (max time)						
BALANCE						
Right Foot Hops (# in 1 min)						
Left Foot Hops (# in 1 min)						
OR						
Right Foot Standing (max time)						
Left Foot Standing (max time)						
NOTES						

At this point you have been consistently exercising, and you move around as much as possible every day to get in your steps. In this phase the workouts get a little more advanced and a little bit longer. The bonus is that longer workouts contribute more to your 10,000 steps, so it may even save you time in the long run. Initially the goal was to get you moving regularly. That remains constant, but now you can move with more intensity. The more intense a workout is, the less of it you have to do to reap the same (and in some cases more) benefits.

Many of the exercises in this phase will challenge your balance and your cardiovascular system. Several require using a large number of muscles all at the same time, elevating your need for oxygen, which in turn increases your heart rate and breathing.

> Prepare to sweat a lot and to be pushed a bit further past your comfort zone as it continues to expand.

NEW EQUIPMENT

By now your exercise equipment consists of (at least) a good pair of running shoes, a mat, and some dumbbells. Now consider adding heavier dumbbells—2-5 lbs heavier than what you've been using—and an exercise ball.

ADVANCED WORKOUTS

In the following set of weeks, continue to get in 10,000 steps per day, plus the workouts listed below. To move on to the next phase of exercise, you must complete a minimum of ¾ of all your workouts, without skipping any Killer workouts, and you must maintain 80% compliance to your 10,000 steps too. Adjust your calendar according to your schedule, but remember to keep all the workouts in the same order!

SAMPLE ADVANCED WORKOUT CALENDAR

WEEK	MON	TUE	WED	THU	FRI	SAT	SUN
1	A*	SI #2		SI #3	K #5		
2	K #5	SI #2		SI #3	K# 5		
3	K #6	SI #2	K #5	SI #3	K# 6		
4	K #6	SI #2	K #5	SI #3	K #6		
5	SP #3	SI #2	K #6	SI #3	SP #3		
6	SP #3	SI #2	K #6	SI #3	SP #3		

* While the days do not need to be exact, add the workouts *in this precise order* to your calendar.

Killer #5

Don't forget to warm up and cool down!
Take a 1 minute break in between each set.

Complete *2 sets of series one* and then *2 sets of series two*.

SERIES ONE

(COMPLETE 2 SETS OF FULL SERIES)

EXERCISE	REPS	WEIGHT
1 - Squat Diagonal Press	10/side	Moderate Weight
2 - Plank Off Ball	30 secs	Body Weight
3 - Side Lunges (Dynamic)	12/side	Moderate Weight
4 - Ball Pass	10 reps	Body Weight

SERIES TWO

(COMPLETE 2 SETS OF FULL SERIES)

EXERCISE	REPS	WEIGHT
1 - Transition Lunges	30 secs/side	Body or Light Weight
2 - Frog Planks	8/side	Body Weight
3 - Oblique Crunch Off Ball	12/side	Body Weight

Workout Complete!

Killer #6

Don't forget to warm up and cool down!
Take a 1 minute break in between each set.

Complete *2 sets of series one* and then *2 sets of series two*.

SERIES ONE
(COMPLETE 2 SETS OF FULL SERIES)

EXERCISE	REPS	WEIGHT
1 - Jump Squats	15 reps	Body Weight
2 - Plank with Alternating Row	8/side	Light Weight
3 - Walking Front Lunge with Rotation	12/side	Light Weight
4 - Single Leg Lateral Raise	10/side	Light to Moderate Weight

SERIES TWO
(COMPLETE 2 SETS OF FULL SERIES)

EXERCISE	REPS	WEIGHT
1 - Side Plank with Arm Rotations	10/side	Body Weight
2 - Mid Row (Palms Facing Upward)	12 reps	Moderate Weight
3 - Knee to Elbow Pushups	10 reps	Body Weight

Workout Complete!

Super Pump #3

Don't forget to warm up and cool down!

Complete 2 sets of this series
with a 1 minute break in between each set.

EXERCISE	REPS	WEIGHT
1 - Plank with Alternating Row	30 seconds	Light Weight
2 - Jump Squats	30 seconds	Body Weight
3 - Skipping	30 seconds	Body Weight
4 - Plank Off Ball	30 seconds	Body Weight
5 - Squat Diagonal Press	30 seconds	Light to Moderate Weight
6 - Mid Row (Palms Facing Upward)	30 seconds	Light to Moderate Weight

Workout Complete!

Sweaty Intervals #2

Don't forget to warm up and cool down!
Do as many reps of each exercise as you can in each round.
Each round consists of 30 seconds of exercise followed by a 30 second break.

Go as FAST as you can without compromising good technique.

EXERCISE	ROUNDS	WEIGHT
1 - Jacks	3	Body Weight
2 - High Knees	3	Body Weight
3 - Weighted Punches	3	Light Weight
4 - Wide Jump Squats/Low Jacks	4	Body Weight

Workout Complete!

Sweaty Intervals #3

Don't forget to warm up and cool down!
Do as many reps of each exercise as you can in each round.
Each round consists of 30 seconds of exercise followed by a 30 second break.

Go as FAST as you can without compromising good technique.

EXERCISE	ROUNDS	WEIGHT
1 - Jacks	2	Body Weight
2 - High Knees	2	Body Weight
3 - Weighted Punches	2	Light Weight
4 - Wide Jump Squats/Low Jacks	3	Body Weight
5 - 180 Degree Squats	4	Body Weight
6 - Jumping Jack Planks	4	Body Weight

Workout Complete!

This phase is no joke. It is intense and definitely feels advanced! I felt like I was doing cardio all the time. There are a lot of abdominal exercises in this phase too, which I liked doing because they made me feel like I was "spot reducing" my stomach. Ang said that wasn't really how it worked—the exercises made the muscles stronger, but that didn't isolate the fat-burning potential to the one area.

For my first workout in this phase (Killer #5), I Skyped with Ang. I was feeling quite nervous to workout with her because it had been nearly six weeks of work trips that kept me having to workout on my own. I'm not saying I did not push myself when I was away, but you have no idea what it is like to workout with Ang . . . that's a whole different story.

I had my home gym all set up in the bedroom again with a few new pieces of equipment that included heavier dumbbells and an exercise ball. The computer rang and there in front of me was that grin again. Here we go!

The workout started off not too bad. What I mean is that by the end of the second series I was still standing and had not puked on the floor. The squat diagonal press was kicking my butt, but I liked it because I figured it would help my golf game. Then came the plank off the ball . . . a nightmare I don't want to dwell on (but get used to it, because it's in both the Killer #5 and Super Pump #3 workouts!). The side lunges were particularly awkward and made me feel like a human wishbone—I thought I was going to rip my crotch wide open! Ang said she had seen it happen only once before. "It was a quick surgery, so not to worry." What a smart ass . . . I have no idea where she gets it.

By the time we got to the transition lunges, I was feeling that very familiar urge to "blow my nose."

> It felt like an eternity, but finally the words I love to hear:
> *Workout complete.*

All tallied up, I "blew my nose" a couple of times and "had to fill my water bottle up" only twice during that workout. An improvement from the dozen or so times I had to in other workouts with my favourite daughter. Later, I celebrated with a beer (every win needs to be celebrated). Rock on!

On my own, the running was starting to get really good—I could make it three kilometres without stopping! I was so excited to tell Ang. She was always a long-distance runner and would buy T-shirts in large as gifts for me from her races. She was so proud when she found out and we decided that our goal would be to do the Father's Day run that year. From then on I started texting her about my running conquests.

> This was a really big phase as far as the physical changes went for me. Now, after 18 weeks of dedicated workouts and eating habits that were substantially improved (though not perfect), I was 27 pounds lighter.

I was hitting off the blue tees with my son and son-in-law, even out-driving them every so often! I now know that a lot of what contributed to my weight loss in this phase was the accumulation of nutrition habits, but the intensification of the exercise certainly did not hurt. My nutrition was supporting my weight loss, and my exercise was lining my pocket with golf winnings! I felt twenty years younger.

TERRY'S TIPS

1. Don't take yourself too seriously. You are not going to be perfect at every exercise or during every workout. This is normal. Give yourself a break.

2. Incorporate exercise into other daily routine things. For example, when having wine, I always do a set of ten curls per side before I open the bottle. When I clean the floors, instead of walking around with the vacuum, I lunge forward and back. Rather than bending over to the laundry basket when folding laundry, I squat down to it and back up again. It may seem silly, but all these things really add up!

3. Even if you are doing really well with the exercise, don't lose sight of your nutrition challenges. You need both to make this work.

Exercise will change your life in more ways than you can imagine. I used to think it was just a means to lose weight. It is that, but it also improves your mood and your confidence, and these impact every other aspect of your life in positive ways. I even have more patience now with the dummies on the road that cut me off!

TIME IT RIGHT

*EAT ONE SERVING OF HEALTHY CARBOHYDRATES
AT BREAKFAST AND AFTER WORKOUTS*

8

NUTRITION

REALITY FITNESS NUTRITION AND WORKOUT TRACKER

	Week:								Week:							
	Weight:								Weight:							
Phase	Mon	Tue	Wed	Thu	Fri	Sat	Sun	Mon	Tue	Wed	Thu	Fri	Sat	Sun	80%?
N1: 3L Water															
N2: Breakfast															
N3: Eat 3-4 hrs															
N4: Portions															
N5: Veggies															
N6: Protein															
N7: Fat															
N8: Carbs															
10,000 steps															
Workouts															
Celly Countdown	3	2	1					3	2	1					

Notes:

Carbohydrates are often perceived as comfort foods and sometimes deemed "unhealthy." There have been several diet plans with varying degrees of popularity that cast carbohydrates and grains as pure, fat-inducing evil. This is simply not true. Foods such as pasta, rice, grains, and fruits are important for nutrition, higher energy levels, and better brain function. Your body requires the energy from carbohydrate replenishment to function properly. Carbohydrates are the main energy source for the body and the only direct energy source for the brain. But also, if used strategically, carbohydrates can actually be beneficial for weight loss.

GAME PLAN

Eat one serving of carbohydrates at breakfast and after workouts. With the exception of veggies, eliminate all other carbs at any other time of day.

As soon as your body consumes carbohydrate foods such as fruit or bread, your digestive system breaks down the digestible carbs into sugar, which then enters your blood. Once your blood sugar levels rise, your pancreas produces insulin—a hormone that initiates cellular absorption of blood sugar for energy or storage. As your cells absorb the blood sugar, sugar levels in your bloodstream begin to decline. Once this occurs, your pancreas starts making glucagon—the hormone that signals your liver to start releasing its stored sugar. This coordination between your insulin and your glucagon hormones ensures that the cells in your body, and especially your brain, have a steady supply of blood sugar to function properly. This process works very well provided you do not over consume carbohydrates at a meal. If this occurs, the insulin hormone has no choice but to store the excess carbohydrate as glycogen in your liver and muscles.

Your liver and muscles become saturated with all the glycogen they can handle, leaving the excess carbohydrates with no place to go. They are therefore stored in adipose (fat) tissue, and you gain weight because this overconsumption not only results in the insulin storing the excess carbs, it also prevents your body from using any of your stored body fat for energy.

> Double Whammy! Every time you eat too many carbs (even in a single sitting), not only are you preventing fat stores from being burned, you are adding to the pile.

TYPES OF CARBOHYDRATES

This phase asks you to incorporate carbohydrates into your nutrition program at only the most optimal times of day. For weight loss and better health, timing is critical, but so is the quality of carbohydrates consumed. There are three main types of carbohydrates: sugar, starch, and fibre.

SUGAR
There are two types of sugar. Added sugar or simple sugar (table sugar, or sucrose, for example) is the simplest form of carbohydrate. Nautral sugar occurs as fructose in fruits and vegetables, and as lactose in milk and milk products.

STARCH
Starch is a complex carbohydrate, which means it is made of many sugar units bonded together. Starch occurs naturally in vegetables, grains, and beans.

FIBRE
Fibre is also a complex carbohydrate. Fibre occurs naturally in fruits, vegetables, whole grains, and beans.

> Know that canned beans are likely to contain much more sodium than dried beans. Check the labels!

Your body will thrive if you are consuming carbohydrates that are more of the fibre variety, some of the starch and natural sugar variety, and if you limit the added

GLUTEN

Unless you have been diagnosed by a physician with an autoimmune disorder such as celiac disease, it is unnecessary to omit gluten from your diet. Gluten is a type of protein in wheat and related grains, including barley and rye. It gives elasticity to dough, helping bread rise and keep its shape and often giving the final product a chewy texture. Even if you have celiac disease, it is important to incorporate carbohydrates from non-gluten sources into your diet.

sugar variety. Simple sugar carbs increase your insulin response as a result of the low fibre content, meaning that you use the energy from the simple sugar almost immediately and feel hungry again in a very short period of time. This usually results in overeating. Starch and fibre carbohydrates slow down the insulin response and reduce the blood sugar process that leads to gaining weight and preventing fat loss. Choosing healthy starch or fibre options—such as beans or quinoa—more often than sugar options—such as white bread and cookies—is important for stabilizing insulin levels. If the food is higher in starch or fibre, it takes longer for the body to process it, therefore keeping you feeling more satisfied for a longer period of time.

As mentioned in Nutrition Phase 5, while vegetables are technically carbohydrates, your blood sugar levels do not respond the same to them as fruits, grains, pastas, rice, etc. due to the lower sugar content. For this reason, vegetables do not count as a carbohydrate within this system, and you can eat as many of them as you like (except for potatoes, sweet potatoes, squash, and corn—those starchy veggies still definitely count as carbs).

BEST CARBOHYDRATE SOURCES AND PORTIONS

It's not that carbohydrates are unhealthy; it is that carbohydrates are often eaten in quantities larger than the body needs because they are so delicious! So what, exactly, and how much can you eat, you might be asking. To avoid overeating carbs (and gaining the weight from the excess stored energy), follow these two portion policies when adding carbohydrates to your plate.

1. ½ cup for whatever kind of carbohydrate food.
2. 1 slice of regular sized bread (not a gigantic slice or a really thick slice).

Yes, it's really that simple. But at this stage of the program, sometimes a list is helpful so that you don't need to think too hard about it. Here's a quick list of your best non-vegetable carbohydrate sources.

BEST CARBOHYDRATE SOURCES

Fruits
- Apples (with skin)
- Pears (with skin)
- Berries
- Oranges
- Bananas
- Grapefruits
- Figs
- Dates

Grains
- Bread (whole grain, rye, etc.)
- Oatmeal (steel cut is best)
- Brown or wild rice
- Whole wheat pasta
- Sweet vegetables (squash, sweet potato, turnip, etc.)

For a more comprehensive list of options and portions for your carbohydrates as well as your proteins and fats, check out the chart in Appendix C. You can also find the same chart available to download or print at www.realityfitnessbook.com.

TIMING IS KEY

The timing of your carbohydrate intake has an enormous effect on weight.

> By strategically incorporating carbohydrates into your nutrition plan during certain times of day, you optimize your fat loss results.

IN THE MORNING
When you first wake up in the morning, after having not eaten for several hours, your liver is anxious to receive carbohydrates so it can send sugar to your brain for optimal function. For this reason, it is very important to supply your body with the necessary energy to perform well. It is therefore optimal in terms of fat loss because carbohydrates are readily used at this time of day, so less energy is likely to be stored as fat (provided you eat the correct portion of carbohydrate).

AFTER A WORKOUT

Though insulin is known as the "fat-storage" hormone, it is also very useful for helping your muscles absorb protein after a weight-training workout. As we mentioned in the protein phase, lean muscle burns more calories than fat, so the more muscle you have, the easier it will be to lose weight.

The combination of carbohydrates with protein after a workout helps your body use the protein more efficiently to repair muscle tissue, thereby building more lean muscle.

Only weight training workouts require carbohydrate replenishment.

Cardiovascular activities such as walking, running, sprinting, swimming, etc. do not require carbohydrate replenishment unless you participate in the activities for an hour or longer. You will have ample energy from the other food sources you are eating to complete your walking and other workouts regularly.

I started this program during yet another no-or-low-carb diet phase in the world. When Ang asked me to eat carbs, I was surprised. I had assumed this phase would be about cutting them entirely. Still, after being inundated with information in the media about how carbs were the enemy and the entire reason we were all fat, I was nervous to start playing around with carbs in my diet: incorporating them sometimes and eliminating them at others. I say nervous because while these are foods I really enjoyed incorporating (and it would not take that much arm-twisting for me to add these in at breakfast and after workouts), I was worried that limiting them at all other times of day would land me in the same position as the last time I tried a carb-free diet—starving myself of them until I broke down and binged on every carb I could get my hands on.

The challenge of the phase sounded pretty straightforward, and it was . . . but I was used to having carbohydrate foods at any time I wanted, and to not have them at will was bothersome. Just when I was on a roll with my food planning, Ang stepped in and messed it all up!

> But then I heard the words: "This is extremely helpful for weight loss." My interest in this inconvenience piqued.

"What do you mean 'extremely'?" I asked. Perhaps a bit more discomfort would be worth it.

I needed a day to wrap my head around this challenge. I couldn't help but reflect back to my juicing. My juice was composed of almost all fruit/carbs. Because juicing allowed me to drink more fruits than I could ever actually eat in a sitting, I was consuming carbs in quantities fit for a family of four, not one person! Even worse, I was drinking these all day long. I was so far from this carb habit, yet at the time I genuinely thought I was doing something good for myself. It wasn't until this stage in Ang's plan that I fully understood why my juice diet caused me to gain so much weight. I guess anything in excess will do this.

I started implementing this new phase the next day, and breakfast was actually simple for me—the fruit in my smoothie counted as my carb for that time of day, so I already had that in the bag. On other days, if I had eggs instead, I added in a piece of toast or a banana. Notice that I said "or" because the phase calls for just one carb in the morning, not two. I stuck to it, and I was on a roll!

Next came my morning snack. Crackers with hummus were no longer an option, as I had not done a workout yet, so I dropped the crackers and added in a few veggies. Not my first choice, but acceptable in my mind. My workout was in the afternoon just before lunch, so I could indulge in an open-faced sandwich. Perfect. I was doing this, and it was going great!

Dinner came around and we were having grilled scallops, asparagus and peppers, and herb potatoes. But damn, the potatoes were carbohydrates. This meant I couldn't partake in these. They looked so good though! Oh boy, I realized in that moment, this is not going to be as easy as it seemed earlier in the day. Carbs were usually a big part of dinner in our household. From here on out I would have two choices. 1) I could do my workout before dinner so I could eat the carbs then (and give up sandwiches for lunch) or 2) I could just suck it up and plan dinners from now on that didn't include carbs. I opted for number two most of the time, as this is what fit into my lifestyle.

It sucked sometimes, but not as much as having to buy XL shirts.

Haha! I make it sound like I just jumped right into this and it was no big deal! Let me tell you that it was not that simple. I struggled . . . a lot. I had the protein and vegetables down, thank goodness! But since I could only have one carb in the morning and one after a workout, I struggled with what carb to choose. Wrapping my head around the idea that a piece of fruit is a carb was hard. For some reason I couldn't see how an apple was the same as a piece of bread or a portion of pasta or rice. Then I figured, hey, chips must be a carb. I can start including those! In my heart I knew better, though. I knew I was trying to find a loophole in the program. Ang explained the different types of carbs to me, but I realized I didn't care about the technical stuff and it was starting to overwhelm me. I just needed her to tell me what to eat. I was done trying to figure it out. For me, the chart she made of the choices for carbs was crucial. I didn't have to think about it, and there was no room to manipulate in a treat disguised as a carb for the day. (You can find the same chart in Appendix C)

Eliminating the carbs from my dinners that weren't post-workout was a really hard thing to do, especially when it came time for special dinners with colleagues or friends. It took about a month before I was able to officially pass this phase into the next one. What finally did it was when, like for other phases, I planned my week in advance. Identifying when I was going out for a meal where carbs would definitely be unavoidable allowed me to plan the rest of my week around those moments to give me the best chance at success.

Just so you know, the only carbs that I gave up entirely were white bread and crackers. I didn't have to according to the program, but for me they were huge trigger foods and so I, by my own choice, banished them from the house. I figured I could eat the grainy shit that Ang suggested for more fibre to replace my bread. The crackers I simply gave up, because I could never help eating too many of them. Other than these two omissions, I was still able eat all the carb choices I used to.

TERRY'S TIPS

1. Pay close attention to your portion sizes. It is very easy to add "just a little extra," and indulging can tip the scales in the opposite direction of where you want to go.

2. Choose your carbohydrate wisely. The less processed, the more nutritious and beneficial to your health. Stick to the chart and you can't go wrong.

3. Think about this phase as "earning" your carbohydrates. Every time you do a weight training workout (Killer) or a circuit (Super Pump), you have earned your carbohydrate. Knowing you can follow up with a carb can be a big motivator to exercise!

Carbs are very important for energy and overall health, but we don't need as many as we think. This phase was extremely effective, just like Ang promised. Part of the reason it is so effective is because it controls how often you eat these kinds of foods. Having parameters for carbs made it easier for me to control them. In the end, I felt the most "trim" during this phase of the program. But this phase was also pretty difficult. It took several weeks for me to get into a regular, consistent pattern of following the plan. When I did get the hang it, though, I noticed that my jeans were looser. In one month of adding in this habit, I saw a two-inch decrease in my waist size. I had to buy new pants! And shorts. Shit, it was annoying to have to shop, but kind of rewarding too.

TIMING CELLIES

CELLIES

*GRADUALLY DECREASING, BUT DEFINITELY **NOT** ELIMINATING TREATS*

Part Three

CELLIES

REALITY FITNESS NUTRITION AND WORKOUT TRACKER

	Week:								Week:							
	Weight:								Weight:							
Phase	Mon	Tue	Wed	Thu	Fri	Sat	Sun		Mon	Tue	Wed	Thu	Fri	Sat	Sun	80%?
N1: 3L Water																
N2: Breakfast																
N3: Eat 3-4 hrs																
N4: Portions																
N5: Veggies																
N6: Protein																
N7: Fat																
N8: Carbs																
10,000 steps																
Workouts																
Celly Countdown		2	1						2	1						

Notes:

It's that time again! Yes, we are ramping things up a little more. In this next celly phase you will now track no more than two cellies per week. As you become more advanced with your fitness and nutrition, so do the tips. In this section, we explore the optimal times of day to incorporate your cellies. Before we expand on this further, though, I understand that it is not always realistic to plan this much. But being more knowledge-able and aware can subconsciously affect your decisions for the better.

GAME PLAN

Limit your cellies to two per week.

TIMING YOUR CELLIES

Just like when you eat carbs, there is an ideal time for indulging in your cellies. In a perfect world, you would keep treats to the daytime versus late at night when your body does not have a lot of time to burn off the extra calories.

If you eat treats or extras earlier in the day, you might have a chance to work some of the excess off.

The best time to indulge in a treat is right after a workout. During the post-weight training workout window, a treat stands a greater chance of being used by your muscles instead of being stored as fat. As mentioned in the carbohydrate phase, the combination of carbs (even in treat form) with protein after a workout helps your body use the protein more efficiently to repair muscle tissue, thereby building more lean muscle mass.

Avoid having a carb *and* a celly post-workout unless they are a single item, otherwise you risk blowing all your workout benefits out the window.

Keep in mind, again, that this timing is merely a suggestion. Of course planning cellies around workouts would make it difficult to, for example, enjoy a beer after a long workday with your co-workers. The timing of your cellies is not a requirement of this phase of the program. You are not asked to track when you indulge in a celly, simply that you have.

T-MAN'S STRAIGHT TALK

I told you I'd be honest, right from the beginning. When Ang told me about timing cellies post-workout, I was all over the idea of having that extra "edge." But when it came right down to it—despite knowing how it was more optimal at that time—I just couldn't wrap my head around eating something "bad" immediately after I worked so hard in the gym.

Ha! Isn't it funny how after a workout the drive to eat healthier is strong and I avoid eating treats even though they are likely to be burned off, but on some random Tuesday after a late day of work I can stuff something awesome (i.e. unhealthy) in my mouth and make no connection to how hard I will have to work to burn that off anyway!

I think that's the key right there . . . fitness freaks like Ang who have been doing this forever have the effort/reward formula ingrained into them so they are much less likely to indulge too often. It all goes back to the same thing: practice, practice, and practice. The more you do it, the easier it becomes. I can say that I never did use her timing tip on that one. But that doesn't mean you shouldn't, at least from time to time. I'm sure it works!

What I did have to do, though, was get back to tracking. I thought I was doing really well (and I was), but as the weeks went on I naturally loosened the portion sizes a bit and also stopped tracking as religiously. My old ways wanted to creep back into my life and I was slowly letting it happen. I guess that is how it all starts.

> You begin with the correct portion size, then you decide one day to have "one extra scoop" convincing yourself that it won't make that big of a difference. Then it leads to another extra scoop at the next meal, then an extra snack because you can . . . and then before you know it you have gone back to your old ways and old weight.

It's so easy to let this happen. At the time it seems so insignificant, and if it was only that one extra scoop, it would be. But that is typically not where it stops. Simply put, by this stage of the program I had to re-establish some tracking habits to pay attention to what I was doing so that I did not let it get out of hand. That's why tracking my cellies on paper was eye opening for me, especially at this stage—it helped me put those extras into perspective and to realize that I was definitely eating more of them than I wanted to admit.

For every extra scoop of something, I was adding calories my body did not need and would therefore store as fat. I realized I would have to burn off these extra scoops during exercise to continue to lose weight. It then became a choice: do I want to eat an extra snack because I'm bored or just feel like eating more, and then run an extra fifteen minutes? Or would I rather not add extra running to my workout program? Sometimes I would opt for the extra running, but with my busy schedule that was not very often.

COLOURS & VITAMINS

*EAT AT LEAST THREE COLOURS
OF FOOD AT EVERY MEAL*

9

NUTRITION

REALITY FITNESS NUTRITION AND WORKOUT TRACKER

	Week:							Week:						
	Weight:							Weight:						
	Mon	Tue	Wed	Thu	Fri	Sat	Sun	Mon	Tue	Wed	Thu	Fri	Sat	Sun
Phase														80%?
N1: 3L Water														
N2: Breakfast														
N3: Eat 3-4 hrs														
N4: Portions														
N5: Veggies														
N6: Protein														
N7: Fat														
N8: Carbs														
N9: Colours														
10,000 steps														
Workouts														
Celly Countdown		2	1						2	1				

Notes:

Vitamins and minerals have multiple roles. While they do not provide energy in the way carbs, protein, and fat do, they support your body's normal growth and development. They are essential for your body to perform at its optimal level. Vitamins and minerals:

- help to maintain or boost your immune system,
- keep your bones and nerves strong,
- help your muscles contract and relax properly,
- keep your heart muscles working properly,
- keep fluids balanced in your body, and
- support your eyesight.

GAME PLAN

Eat a minimum of three colours of food every meal; one must be green. The colours must be distinctly different. Having more than three colours is absolutely okay, but different shades of a colour do not count as more than one.

The average person eats only about twenty different types of food on a regular basis. It is not surprising, then, that many people are lacking vital nutrients that support a healthy body. It is easy to stick to a selection of your favourite foods every week, but if you stick to the same ones for too long you are likely going to miss out on important vitamins. Food can also become very mundane. This system is about weight loss, but it is also about overall health and long-term sustainability. Without a variety of foods to choose from, continuing this process for the long term can become difficult. By focusing on the colours of your food you are much more likely to get a variety of nutrients into your diet while avoiding boredom.

VITAMINS & MINERALS

Ensuring a variety of foods, and therefore vitamins and nutrients in your diet, keeps your body guessing! The human body is a clever machine. If you are constantly doing the same thing or eating the same thing, your body finds the most efficient way to handle the situation. By slightly altering the foods you eat once in a while, you'll prevent your body from taking the shortcut (thereby burning fewer calories).These are the 13 essential vitamins: Vitamins A, C, D, E, K, and the B vitamins—thiamine (B1), riboflavin (B2), niacin (B3), pantothenic acid (B5), pyridoxine (B6), biotin (B7), folate (B9), and cobalamin (B12).

Vitamins A, D, E, and K are fat-soluble and are stored in the fatty tissue of the body. The B vitamins are water-soluble and are important to replenish regularly since they are removed from the body through your urine. Vitamin B12 is the only water-soluble vitamin that is stored in the liver.

The body also requires essential minerals for optimal wellness. A balanced diet can help reduce the risk of deficiency in one mineral or another. Essential minerals are divided into two categories and can be found in most fresh foods.

Macrominerals (major minerals): calcium, magnesium, potassium, phosphorus, sodium, sulphur, and chloride.

Microminerals (trace minerals): iron, zinc, iodine, selenium, copper, fluoride, manganese, chromium, molybdenum, nickel, silicon, vanadium, and cobalt.

NUTRIENTS IN COLOUR

You are likely to obtain a wider variety of vitamins and an overall healthier diet if you use colour as your guide in choosing fruits and vegetables. Certainly there is nothing wrong with eating a lot of green vegetables. However, research has suggested that the wider the variety of colour on your plate, the better your nutritional needs are met. Certain colours of foods are higher in specific vitamins. If you opt to eat only red fruits and vegetables, for example, you might miss out on other vitamins found in yellow fruits and veggies. By paying attention to the colours in your meals and incorporating a rainbow on your plate, you will be more likely to boost your vitamin content throughout the week. Still, green is the most important colour of this rainbow.

The reason you are asked to make sure one of your food colours at every meal is green is because green vegetables contain the highest levels of vitamins and minerals, and yet they are often the first vegetables to be skipped.

GREEN VEGETABLES

Sugar snap peas	Cauliflower	Watercress
Zucchini	Collard greens	Cucumber
Green peppers	Turnip greens	Asparagus
Peas	Swiss chard	Beet greens
Green onions	Spinach	Brussels sprouts
Leeks	Mustard greens	Celery
Green beans	Broccoli	Endive
Chinese cabbage	Rapini (broccoli rabe)	Sprouts
Kale	Lettuce	Alfalfa
Arugula	Cabbage	Turnip greens
Butterhead lettuce	Bok choy	

BUILD YOUR RECIPE REPERTOIRE

A great way to integrate a more colourful variety of foods into your diet and to mix up your eating go-tos is by experimenting with new recipes and items you've never tried before. When you're seeking to incorporate different colours, you can be inspired by new cooking ideas and recipes. Now is the time to experiment and build your food palate.

Don't forget about foods from different cultures, different spices, different ingredients—the possibilities are endless!

WEBSITES TO FIND NEW RECIPES

- www.fooducate.com
- www.epicurious.com
- www.mensfitness.com
- www.eatingwell.com
- www.finecooking.com
- www.menshealth.com

Of course there are also several apps where you can find great recipes too. A favourite is Wholesome -Healthy Eating. The app divides foods up by colour and helps you to understand the variety of nutrients you're getting based on what you're eating.

SALADS

Salads are a fantastic way to incorporate several colours of veggies at once. Here's a quick salad formula to make salad creation less intimidating. Remember that having all your ingredients washed, chopped, and in the fridge ready to go will make putting these together even easier.

1. Pick 1-2 types of lettuce or leafy greens (pre-mixed packs of greens are great for saving time)

2. Add two different colours of vegetables (e.g. red peppers, orange carrots) *For extra salad-appeal, use a berry as one of your colours!

3. Add one tablespoon of a chopped, fresh herb (e.g. basil, mint, parsley, dill)

4. Add a protein (e.g. fish, beef, chicken, shrimp, tofu, boiled eggs)

5. Add a healthy fat (e.g. olive oil salad dressing)

MAKE A SOUP

As always, soups are fantastic and a nice addition to any meal. They also present a great opportunity to integrate green into your meal. Here are two delicious green soup recipes.

ZUCCHINI SOUP I NEVER THOUGHT I'D EAT IN MY LIFE AND ACTUALLY SAY I LIKED IT

Ingredients

2 pounds zucchini, trimmed and cut crosswise into thirds
1 ½ tsp salt, divided
¾ cup onion, chopped
2 garlic cloves, chopped
¼ cup olive oil
4 cups water, divided
⅓ cup packed basil leaves

* Equipment: an adjustable blade slicer fitted with ⅛ inch julienne attachment

Directions

1. Julienne skin (only) from half of zucchini with slicer. Toss with ½ teaspoon salt and drain in a sieve until wilted, at least 20 minutes. Coarsely chop remaining zucchini.

2. Cook onion and garlic in oil in a 3- to 4-quarts heavy saucepan over medium-low heat, stirring occasionally, until softened, about 5 minutes. Add chopped zucchini and 1 teaspoon of salt and cook, stirring occasionally, about 5 minutes. Add 3 cups of water and simmer, partially covered, until tender, about 15 minutes.

3. Purée soup with basil in two batches in a blender (use caution when blending hot liquids) or in the pot using an immersion blender.

4. Bring remaining cup of water to a boil in a small saucepan and blanch julienned zucchini for 1 minute. Drain in a sieve set over a bowl so that you can use the liquid to thin the soup if necessary.

5. Top bowls of soup with julienned zucchini. Season soup with salt and pepper to taste.

BROCCOLI SOUP EVEN MY DAD WILL EAT

Ingredients

1 tbsp olive oil

1 large onion, chopped

3 garlic cloves, chopped

2 10-oz packages chopped frozen broccoli, thawed

1 potato, peeled and chopped

4 cups chicken broth

¼ tsp ground nutmeg

salt and pepper to taste

Directions

1. Heat olive oil in a large saucepan and sauté onion and garlic until tender.

2. Mix in broccoli, potato, and chicken broth. Bring to a boil. Reduce heat and then simmer for about 15 minutes, until the vegetables are tender.

3. With a hand mixer or in a blender, purée the mixture until smooth.

4. Return to the saucepan and reheat. Season with nutmeg, salt, and pepper.

And just like that, here I was. Almost the end of mastering my new eating habits. I began to realize around this point that not only was I losing weight, but I was really gaining a sense of what it was like to eat and be healthy. The entire process was coming together. Maybe it was because I knew I had only a few weeks left before "completing" the program, but I also think it had a lot to do with how my body felt—as though I was doing a good job feeding it. I was light. I had more energy than I could remember ever having.

So the next phase from Ang was to incorporate three colours of food into every meal, and one of them had to be green, always. Why green? I asked. Ang explained that green veggies were the ones that contained the most vitamins and nutrients. Even calcium!

> Go figure, the calcium I was worried about losing from all but eliminating milk from my diet early on would now be replaced by broccoli. Amazing!

Turns out I was already completing this ritual, more or less. When I had my smoothie in the morning it included red raspberries, white protein powder, and green spinach, so I was doing well there. At one point I tried to switch it up and experimented by adding celery to the mix. How it can make a smoothie taste so bad is beyond my comprehension. You don't realize how strong a flavour celery has until you add it to your morning protein shake. I highly recommend you don't do this. It's awful! Stick to the spinach. When I opted for eggs in the morning, I used to only add tomatoes to the side of my plate. That's only two colours (white for the eggs and red for the tomatoes), so I started to include a handful of cucumber for a bit of green.

Incorporating the tri-colour habit into lunches and dinners was also easy. I just focused more attention on having two different vegetables at each meal rather than having two handfuls of the same vegetable. For greens, I added in one of the following at every meal: cucumber, broccoli, spinach, zucchini, or some sort of lettuce for a salad. I wasn't a fan of green veggies, but if I thought of the green vegetable as my "vitamin" instead, then I was more likely to suck it up and eat it. Sometimes I ended up adding the green vegetable as a fourth colour.

> This phase helped me realize that I used to eat the same things day in and day out.

Again, this phase was not difficult, it just required a bit more planning. Tomatoes and orange bell peppers were my default veggies. Of course there was nothing wrong with these, it was just I knew I was missing out on some vitamins that were not in my repertoire. I needed to start including new foods into my diet not necessarily just for appearance, but for the variety of vitamins. Not to mention I was starting to get bored in Tomato Land, and those fried foods and sweets that I was limiting were starting to look more and more tempting again. By focusing on the addition of new colours to my meals, I would keep to my program plan and continue to get healthier and healthier by the meal!

> I had to mix it up if I was going to stay true to my goal.
> Attempting one new recipe a week was the solution.

Every Friday I would search online or in our cookbooks for a new recipe that incorporated a different colour of food. This way I was building a database of go-to meals I could make. Over the months I found several recipes that were easy, healthy, and provided some great variety. There were a few duds along the way. I made a few soups that tasted like absolutely nothing. Seriously, nothing! These recipes have not been included in this book. But at the end of Nutrition Phase 10 there's a few winners from my now significantly expanded recipe database.

While this phase was great for breaking routine, I'd like to add that my wife was really impressed—both with my new physique and with my cooking that got better and better as I kept up with this phase.

> They say the way to a man's heart is through his stomach.
> Turns out it can be the same way to a woman's heart too!

TERRY'S TIPS

1. Don't overcomplicate the tri-colour phase. All you need is a green vegetable and then two other colours. Your protein is likely to be brown or white (conveniently not the colour of most vegetables), so all you have to do is add one more vegetable that is any colour but green. Done!

2. Stick to one new recipe a week. Attempting a full week of new recipes can be overwhelming, but one at a time on a weekly basis can be a fun way to switch it up and expand your taste buds.

3. When you find the recipe you're going to attempt, take a screen shot or a photo of the ingredient list with your phone. That way you have the grocery list handy at the store.

4. For easy variety, switch out a single ingredient in one of your routine meals. Sometimes all it takes is a small substitution and suddenly you have a new supper! Replace the dill pickles with jalapeños in your ground turkey and change the taste of your burgers or bolognese. Maybe that doesn't change the colour, but it sure does switch things up.

5. Green salsa. I put that shit on everything! Behold, the recipe that changed everything for me.

TERRY'S GREEN SALSA

Ingredients

8 tomatillos, husked
3 shallots
2 garlic cloves, peeled
1 4-oz can green chilli peppers, chopped
¼ cup fresh cilantro, chopped
1 fresh jalapeño pepper, seeded
salt to taste

Directions

1. In a food processor, place tomatillos, shallots, garlic, green chili peppers, cilantro, jalapeño pepper, and salt.

2. Using the pulse setting, coarsely chop.

3. Transfer to a serving dish. Cover and chill in the refrigerator until serving.

FOOD LABELS

CONSUME FRESH FOODS AND ONLY THOSE PROCESSED FOODS THAT COMPLY WITH THE LABEL READING TEST

10

NUTRITION

REALITY FITNESS NUTRITION AND WORKOUT TRACKER

	Week:								Week:							
	Weight:								Weight:							
Phase	Mon	Tue	Wed	Thu	Fri	Sat	Sun	Mon	Tue	Wed	Thu	Fri	Sat	Sun	80%?
N1: 3L Water															
N2: Breakfast															
N3: Eat 3-4 hrs															
N4: Portions															
N5: Veggies															
N6: Protein															
N7: Fat															
N8: Carbs															
N9: Colours															
N10: Natural Food															
10,000 steps															
Workouts															
Celly Countdown		2	1						2	1					

Comments:

Healthy eating can be confusing at times. One minute we are told to eat Food X for some health benefit and then the next day not to eat Food X for some new reason that hurts our health. But there is one common theme to nearly every nutrition or diet plan out there: eat food from nature, a.k.a. real food. Food from nature is simply better for your body than food that has been chemically enhanced or altered in a factory. Consider the following:

- An apple picked from a tree.
- An apple cut up and put into a plastic container (maybe with a dipping sauce).
- An apple puréed and mixed with other fruit to make a chewy bar.
- An apple puréed, sugar added and made into apple chews.
- An apple squeezed, sugar added and made into juice.
- Apple flavour added (but actually there is no apple).

This is just one example of how we can take a simple, natural food and turn into something so far removed from what it once was. The apple is nutritious, easy to pack, and even costs less than the other options. The latter options provide your body with little to no nutrition and might even be harmful over the long-term due to added sugars.

GAME PLAN

Eat only natural foods and processed goods that meet the label requirements.

It is not as convenient all the time, but incorporating fresh foods is essential to your well-being, and relying on pre-made foods compromises your health in the long-term. While processed foods are fast, they often lack nutritional value and are high in fat, sugar, salt, and calories—and it's not even that they need these ingredients for the sake of increasing shelf life. Foods such as crackers, cereals, chips, and granola bars are scientifically designed to increase the amount of food you eat by calculating the exact salt-to-sugar ratio that leaves you wanting more and eating more. This equates to you buying more of their product, and while that's fantastic for their bottom line, it's not so great for your bottom. In the short term, you might be saving time by eating quick, easy, packaged meals. But consider how many hours you have to put in at the gym to work that off—in the end, you're not saving time at all.

SUGAR AND SODIUM MAXIMUMS

Most people love salty and sweet foods. Unfortunately, a diet that is high in sodium and sugar is harmful to our waistlines and increases our risk of heart disease, diabetes, and high blood pressure. You can reach or exceed the recommended daily allowance of sugar and/or salt by consuming even a single packaged food item!

Many health organizations, such as the Heart and Stroke Foundation, recommend 2300 mg a day of sodium for most individuals. For those with high blood pressure, chronic kidney disease, diabetes, or those who are over 51 years of age or African American, 1500 mg per day of sodium is recommended.

$$2300 \text{ mg sodium} = 5 \text{ ml} = 1 \text{ tsp}$$

For added sugars, The American Heart Association recommends the equivalent of 9 teaspoons of sugar a day (6 teaspoons for women).

$$150 \text{ calories of sugar} = 36 \text{ g} = 9 \text{ tsp}$$

THE LABEL TEST

Food labels can make you crazy by making you feel like you are doing everything wrong. Worse, they can sometimes make you feel like you're doing everything right, even though you might not be. There are a number of things to fixate on when it comes to food and food labels: ingredients, calories, fat content, trans fat content, saturated fat content, sugar, sodium, calcium, iron, vitamin C, fibre . . . it goes on and on and on. It's easier to just avoid it all by sticking to natural, unprocessed foods.

All this said, there are still plenty of nutritious options that fall into the category of "processed" goods. If you are going to choose one, make sure the processed food is suitable by using the following tests to evaluate it.

TEST #1: FEWER THAN TEN
If there are more than ten ingredients on the label, put the food down.

TEST #2: CAN YOU PRONOUNCE IT?
If there are fewer than ten ingredients, but you can't pronounce them all or do not know what one or more of the ingredients is, put the food down.

TEST #3: SUGAR
If the serving size's total grams of sugar is more than 5 g, put the food down.

TEST #4: SODIUM
If the serving size label reads sodium over 5% DV or over 120 mg, put the food down.

Check the serving size! Often the package size is more than the serving size stated on the label.

If your food choice passes all of the above tests, it is considered an acceptable addition to your diet as a snack or part of a meal. You might be surprised at how limiting these parameters are. You will be putting a lot of foods back on the shelves and opting to buy more fresh foods if only to avoid the frustration!

Of course there are times when eating packaged goods is, for one reason or another, your only option, or maybe it's a celly! This is the last nutrition phase of the program. Maybe you will or maybe you won't be able to knock it off the list. Eliminating packaged foods entirely and for good, for most people, is unrealistic. But becoming more aware of added sugars and salts—and reading and understanding labels—is a huge step forward toward your health. You'll inevitably begin to make better choices for your body in the long-term.

Know that you don't have to give up everything to be considered healthy!

T-MAN'S STRAIGHT TALK

By this time I was feeling pretty darn good about my efforts. I was able to sit down at every meal and feel confident that I was eating a plate of food that would nourish my body, make me feel satisfied, and keep me feeling trim. It had been weeks of phasing in the habits to make them just that, habit. Then I noticed that I was beginning to get lured in by certain "health" products at the grocery store, and I wasn't necessarily sure I was doing the right thing by eating them. The reality was, I didn't know what to look for on the food label to understand fully if the product was actually healthy or good for me.

I had heard the term "processed" a lot on TV, but I never really understood what it meant. I figured only foods like chips and chocolate bars were considered processed, and they were full of fat, so they made you fat. Boy, was I ever wrong.

I knew that junk food was not good for your health, but I had no idea that many of the foods I was eating—things I never considered junk food, like some yogurts or most granola bars—were also unhealthy because of all the added salt, sugar, and chemicals.

> Here I was thinking my bars and yogurts were helping me to be more healthy, but in reality, they were making the problem worse! I felt deceived. Tricked. Manipulated!

"This is why it is important to educate yourself on what good nutrition looks like and how to read food labels," said Ang. When she explained the amount of salt and sugar added into processed foods—even to the ones claiming to be healthy—and then asked me to avoid packaged products that didn't follow her very strict guidelines, I began to worry again that there would be nothing for me to eat. I was especially worried for my snacks. It would be easy to eat natural foods for meals because of the previous habits ingrained in me already, but I tended to rely on packaged goods for my snacks because they were easy and added variety to my days. Was I going to have to give up my trail mix bars, my granola cereal and yogurt, my peanut butter, my pepperoni sticks, and my cinnamon spice oatmeal? "Eat foods that grew on a farm, not in a factory," she said. "If the food was not around 100 years ago, don't buy it."

> I began to picture myself churning my own butter. This was not what I wanted for my life.

I understood nutritious food was important for my health, but I did not have the time or the desire to start making my own cheese. Panic was setting in. Could I eat bread anymore? It came in a plastic bag. Did that make it processed? Ang said yes and that while it would be best to make my own, there were still store breads I could eat. I think my reaction indicated there was no freaking way that was happening. Could I still eat my protein bars? Ang said yes, as long as the ingredient list was all foods that I could pronounce, and granted the sodium and sugar levels weren't above the allowable limit. I went to check the boxes right away and realized that every single bar I had in the fridge was full of ingredients that left me clueless. What the hell is potassium sorbate? It sounds like sorbet to me, but I am doubtful that it's as tasty. How about soy lecithin, propyl gallate, BHA, or sodium benzoate? This was when the meaning of the word "processed" really clicked for me. The names of these ingredients sounded like something made in a laboratory. Then it occurred to me . . . that's exactly where they were made! These were not foods, they were chemicals.

> I began to understand that the less packaging a food had,
> the better and healthier it was.

But there were still some packaged foods that I wanted to eat and that were a regular part of my diet. Yogurt, cheese, butter, bread, pasta, milk. I didn't want to find alternatives for these all! But reading the labels on all the foods in my fridge turned out to be depressing.

Because Ang was in Canada and I was in the States, she couldn't join me in person on a grocery store tour. We opted to Face Time as our next best option. I carried Ang around on my phone as I walked through the supermarket and pointed out foods I still wanted to eat on a regular basis. We started at my favourite: the dairy section. Looking at the milk, my heart dropped. It had too much sugar per serving. How could milk not fit the bill? But Ang intervened and said it was okay to have skim, 1%, or even 2%. I just had to adjust the serving size to be a bit smaller than that on the label (to 250 mL) so that the milk fit into the guidelines. Problem solved! I could still have my milk. For cheese it was the same thing. Buy a good quality cheese that was made of dairy, not plastic, and keep the serving size to about that of two dice (I had already practised this with the fats phase). For yogurt, I must have looked at about fifteen different options before one eventually met Ang's criteria. I was amazed at how much sugar was added to them! Almost all yogurts were a no-go with the exception of the Greek style, unflavoured varieties.

Next we were off to the bread section. I was never a big bread eater, but a sandwich is nice once in a while when you don't have a lot of time to cook a meal. Ang walked me through the label reading again, starting with the ingredients. If there were any mystery ingredients, I put it down and moved on to the next option. Once I had a bread that was full of ingredients I understood, we looked at the nutrition label and went through the steps. It turned out that most of the grainier/seedier breads were all pretty good options. Thank goodness, I could buy bread still and was not going to have to make my own. There are some things I'm willing to do, and then there are some things I'm just not pumped for. Would I rather golf or stay home and make bread? Seriously.

IS IT GOOD?

This may not sound very technical, but here are a few things that helped me understand what I could eat to maintain my nutrition level (which by this point was starting to be pretty awesome).

1. If the food is grown from a plant or tree outside, it is good.

2. If the food comes from an animal on a farm, it is good.

3. If the food has an ingredient list with words/foods I can pronounce and I know what they are, it is good.

4. The fewer the ingredients, the better.

The last sections we visited in the supermarket were the a with all the snack options. If you want to skip this next paragraph and save yourself from the detailed version of this depressing information, go right ahead. The short version of the story is: almost every single snack food you look at—even if it says natural or healthy or heart healthy or touts swanky ingredients like goji berries or omega 3, blah blah blah—it's almost certain you'll have to put it down. I'm telling you, just save yourself the torture and shop the perimeter of the store where all the real foods are. I picked up no less than thirty products (I'm persistent, as you know by now) and not a single one met the criteria! Not. A. Single. One. In fact, most were so far off the mark that Ang just started laughing at the absurdity. I didn't get it. It must have been some weird gym-guru trainer humour that only they get. She was almost hysterical a few times, but I didn't think it was that funny. Actually, I didn't think it was funny at all! It pissed me off. How can companies put "foods" on the shelf like this and say it's food? And even more, how can they market it as healthy? I realized I was going to have to take my snacks into my own hands. I would make my own bars, damn it!

It took a while to find foods that worked, and in the process I learned that reading food labels is extremely disappointing. But with a little practice and several trips to the store, I was able to build a list of items that were good to eat and ones to avoid.

Bottom line is if the label didn't match the requirements, I put the food down and kept looking. If I was unable to find an item that matched, I left without it.

It has been a few years now since I learned how to read labels, and I can assure you that I have only come across a handful of processed snack products that meet the guidelines. I did not realize how many packaged goods were actually poor choices. I thought I was perhaps reading the labels wrong initially because I could not find a food that was okay to buy according the rules. Unfortunately I was reading the labels correctly. This is just what we are faced with . . . a lot of high sugar, high salt, processed foods. And yet, it's impossible to make all your own stuff, so sometimes you have to buy processed goods. But I always feel empowered to check and see what I am putting into my body. I can be confident and educated in my choices (even if sometimes I make the conscious choice to eat a snack every now and then that doesn't meet the guidelines). Just trust that fresh is always best, and the fewer labels you read, the better the food you are feeding your body. Darn it, I think I finally understand what this healthy eating thing is all about. I think I might have just been hit by lightning . . . was that a crack of thunder I just heard?

TERRY'S TIPS

1. Avoid food with labels as much as possible by shopping the perimeter of the grocery store. This is where the healthiest options are. Even better, visit a farmers' market for fresh foods. It is a nice way to get out, meet the farmers in your area, and buy the best foods while supporting your local economy!

2. Do not trust the marketing claims on the front of packaged goods. It can be very tempting to pick up pre-packaged "health" foods. Especially when they are labelled with fancy health-wording like "wholesome" or "natural." The box might have a picture of fresh foods on a sunny farm next to some ripped dude, but it's all marketing bullshit! Certain health check logos are images merely purchased by companies with loose terms as to what qualifies the foods as "healthy." Always check the labels yourself.

3. Don't bend the label rules. Even if the item you're considering is close to the recommended sugar and sodium numbers, it still does not count. Setting boundaries is important, otherwise it becomes a slippery slope. 5 g of sugar to 6 g of sugar to 8 g of sugar . . .

4. Learn to make some of your favourite packaged goods at home. Protein bars, granola bars, potato chips, pizza, etc. can all be made at home with healthier, natural ingredients.

5. Here are a few recipes for my favourite foods I used to buy as packaged goods. These foods are certainly not "health" foods, but at least they are made with real food ingredients—not chemicals—and have some nutritional value to them.

MORE GREAT RECIPES

LEEK AND FETA FRITTATA

Ingredients

1 tbsp olive oil

2 large leeks, thinly sliced

1 garlic clove, crushed

1 small red pepper, thinly sliced

8 eggs, beaten

1/3 cup milk

150 g feta cheese, crumbled (I like to buy the pre-crumbled variety)

1/4 cup parmesan cheese, grated

2 tbsp fresh parsley, chopped

1/4 cup extra parmesan cheese to top

Directions

1. Grease a medium-sized square cake tin and line with parchment paper.

2. Heat oil in a pan and cook leeks, garlic, and red pepper just until soft and lightly browned. Cool.

3. Combine leek mixture with beaten eggs, milk, cheeses, and parsley. Mix the ingredients well.

4. Pour mixture into prepared tin and sprinkle top with extra cheese. Cook in a 350°F oven for about 40 minutes. Cool in the cake tin. Cut into squares to serve.

TURKEY VEGGIE MEATLOAF CUPS

Ingredients

2 cups zucchini, coarsely chopped

1 red bell pepper, coarsely chopped

1 pound extra lean ground turkey

1 egg

spice any way you like
   (just a little salt and pepper is even nice)

Directions

1. Preheat oven to 400°F. Spray 20 muffin cups with cooking spray.

2. Mix all of the ingredients together and press evenly into muffin tins.

3. Bake in the preheated oven until juices run clear, about 25 minutes. Internal temperature of a muffin measured by an instant-read meat thermometer should be at least 160°F. Let stand 5 minutes before serving.

MEXICAN TORTILLA SOUP

Ingredients

tsp olive oil, divided

12 ounces skinless, boneless chicken breast, trimmed and diced

1 cup onion, chopped

1 cup green bell pepper, chopped

2 garlic cloves, minced (1 teaspoon)

¾ tsp ground cumin

¾ tsp chilli powder

2 14-oz cans low-sodium chicken broth

1 19-oz can diced tomatoes, undrained

⅓ cup fresh cilantro, chopped

½ cup shredded Mexican blend cheese

6 lime wedges (about 1 ½ limes)

Directions

1. Heat 1 tsp of oil in a non-stick Dutch oven over medium-high heat. Add the chicken and cook, stirring often, 3-4 minutes or until browned. Remove the chicken to plate and cover.

2. In the same Dutch oven, heat the remaining tsp of oil on medium-high. Add the onion, bell pepper, and garlic. Cook, stirring often, 5 minutes or until softened. Stir in cumin, chili powder, broth, and tomatoes. Bring to a boil. Reduce heat and simmer for 5 minutes.

3. Return the chicken and juices to the Dutch oven and simmer 3 minutes or until heated through. Stir in cilantro.

4. Ladle soup into serving bowls and top with 1 tbsp of cheese. Serve hot, with a lime wedge on the side.

NUTRITIOUS ENERGY BAR

Ingredients

2.5 cups rolled oats

¼ cup sesame seeds

2 tbsp almonds, chopped

1 tbsp cashews, chopped

1 tbsp ground flaxseed (optional)

½ cup water

¾ cup almond butter

½ cup honey

1 cup mixed dried fruit, roughly chopped
  (e.g. raisins, apricots)

a pinch of salt

Directions

1. Preheat the oven to 350°F.

2. Combine oats, seeds, nuts, and flaxseed. Spread evenly onto a sheet pan and bake until light brown, about 10 to 12 minutes. Pour the mixture into a large bowl.

3. Boil water in a medium saucepan and remove it from heat. Stir in almond butter and honey, and set the mixture over medium-low heat. Stir constantly until the mixture thickens and pulls away from the sides, about 2 minutes.

4. Mix the fruit and salt into the almond butter mixture, then immediately pour into the bowl with the grains. Using a rubber spatula, stir until the grains are evenly coated.

5. Grease an 8 x 8 inch baking pan with cooking spray, transfer the mixture to the pan and press it into a uniform ½-inch thickness. Move the pan to the refrigerator and allow it to chill for at least two hours.

6. Cut into 1½-inch by 1¼-inch bars. Serve immediately or wrap individually in plastic wrap. Bars will keep for two days at room temperature or four days refrigerated. They can also be frozen to last even longer!

HEALTHIER (BUT STILL TASTY) BUFFALO CHICKEN WINGS

Ingredients

½ cup all-purpose flour

¼ tsp paprika

¼ tsp cayenne pepper

¼ tsp salt

10 chicken wings

2 tbsp butter

¼ cup hot sauce

1 garlic clove, minced

1 dash ground black pepper

Directions

1. Preheat oven to 400°F.

2. Mix together flour, paprika, cayenne pepper, and salt in a small bowl. Place chicken wings in a large dish and sprinkle flour mixture over them until well coated. Place on baking sheet and refrigerate for one hour, uncovered.

3. Bake wings in preheated oven until no longer pink at the bone and juices run clear, about 15 minutes per side.

4. Combine butter, hot sauce, pepper, and garlic in a small saucepan over low heat. Cook and stir until butter is melted and mixture is well blended, about 3 minutes. Place chicken wings in serving bowl and add hot sauce mixture, mixing well.

SWEET POTATO FRIES

Ingredients

4 medium sweet potatoes, peeled and sliced

6 tbsp olive oil

2 tbsp brown sugar (optional)

1 tsp cajun pepper seasoning

a pinch of salt

Directions

1. Preheat oven to 375°F.

2. Place sweet potatoes, olive oil, brown sugar, cajun seasoning, and salt in a large resealable plastic bag. Shake to coat potatoes evenly. Transfer potatoes to a baking dish and spread evenly.

3. Bake in preheated oven, flipping occasionally, until sweet potatoes are tender, about one hour.

REALITY FITNESS

SUSTAINABILITY PHASE

KEEPIN' IT OFF

MAINTAINING YOUR NEW FITNESS
AND NUTRITION HABITS

Sustainability

HEALTH

REALITY FITNESS ASSESSMENT TRACKING FORM

	BUILDING	INTENSIFY	ADVANCED	SUSTAINABILITY		
DATE OF ASSESSMENT						
TIME OF DAY						
BODY COMPOSITION						
Weight						
Neck						
Shoulders						
Chest						
Waist						
Hips						
Right Arm						
Right Leg						
CARDIOVASCULAR FITNESS						
1.5 mile run time						
OR						
1.0 mile walk time						
MUSCULAR ENDURANCE						
Squats (# in 1 minute)						
Pushups Off Toes (max #)						
OR						
Pushups Off Knees (max #)						
Plank off Elbows (max time)						
BALANCE						
Right Foot Hops (# in 1 min)						
Left Foot Hops (# in 1 min)						
OR						
Right Foot Standing (max time)						
Left Foot Standing (max time)						
NOTES						

A question my dad asked when he was approaching his ideal body weight was: how long do I have to do this program for? It was a fair question, but one that concerned me. It sounded like he was thinking that there was an end to the program. The point of *Reality Fitness* is to build a new lifestyle, one that you can continue for the rest of your life. My hasty response? FOREVER. What I should have said and later followed up with was: ideally forever, but with some forgiveness in there so you can still lead the social lifestyle you enjoy.

There've been a lot of changes for you lately, and you might be feeling tired of it all! Maybe you're ready for a break, and that's totally understandable and normal. Nobody can push harder/faster/more for the rest of their life and not burn out physically, mentally, or both. You've already given months of dedication (maybe not perfection, but consistent effort).

Weight loss really is all about calories in not exceeding calories out. Whatever method you use to accomplish this—low carb, marathon running, low fat, no sugar, etc.—as long as you don't eat more than you burn, you will lose weight. But eliminating certain food groups or taking all the things you love out of your daily diet forever would feel like deprivation and would be kind of depressing.

> So, where is the line between weight loss maintenance and still being able to live your life?

Here's how to find that balance once you've come to the point in the program where you've reached your target.

DECIDE YOUR BODY WEIGHT THRESHOLD

Weight ups and downs are normal. Decide how much you are willing to gain—and then ultimately lose—from time to time. This threshold gives you permission to loosen things up for a while on vacation or during an off week. But once you reach that number, know that you have a standard for yourself, and commit to getting back on the program. Everyone will have a different number. You decide what your threshold number is (and know that about every eight pounds equals a pant size).

> Your threshold is not a number you Google. It is a number that you feel good in. You feel healthy and energetic. You like the way your clothes fit, and you are more confident.

REINCORPORATING MORE CELLIES PER WEEK

How many cellies can you incorporate into your week while maintaining your weight within your decided range? This is trial and error. For most, three to four cellies tends to work well.

> If you overdo it one week, then the next week reel yourself in a bit.

The key is to be aware of how many you are having. It is as soon as you lose track of your habits and what you are consuming that sneaky pounds creep back on. Always be aware of what you are ingesting. If it's 12 beers in one night, so be it. At least you know and can counteract that in the following days to keep yourself in check.

CHEATING

Plan for a cheat day once in a while. Yes, I said cheat. Sometimes you just need to take a break from tracking, from everything. Sometimes you need to blow your celly count for the week just because. Take one day a month and eat whatever you want. The caveat here (of course you knew there would be one)—only have this cheat day if you have been at least 80% compliant with the habits the previous six days. You have to earn the cheat day. And maybe be sure to include a weight-training workout on that day too! Okay, I see that I'm already taking the fun out of this . . . I'll stop now.

TAKING A WORKOUT BREAK

If you want (and only if you want) you can opt for a week or two of maintenance training. You can tone the workouts down a bit in intensity (lighter workouts—no intervals and maybe more activity workouts vs. gym workouts like paddle boarding instead of running) and/or you can decrease the number of workouts per week (three or four workouts a week instead of five or six). This break can rejuvenate you physically and mentally. At some point (usually every six months or so) a two-week recovery period can really benefit.

> It's important to have parameters around the break, and taking time off from the gym completely is not recommended.

Make sure you write down what your break period is going to look like. When will it start, and when will it end? Where will you get your activity in and how? Once it's written down, stick to it.

SUSTAINABILITY WORKOUTS

Whether or not you take a break, it's important to continue to switch up your workouts. The following workouts are meant to keep you going on your fitness journey and will, once again, attempt to push you out of your comfort zone (but maybe you're used to that by now). The exercises are more advanced and incorporate more strength, more coordination, more stamina, and more attention to maintaining good technique in order to get the most of the exercises.

Your exercise technique must continue to be the priority. If you find you are unable to complete all of the repetitions of an exercise without losing your form, take a short break and then keep going. Taking short breaks of 30 seconds or less can make a big difference in your ability to finish a set properly.

SAMPLE SUSTAINABILITY WORKOUT CALENDAR

WEEK	MON	TUE	WED	THU	FRI	SAT	SUN
1	A*	SI #3		SI #4	K #7		
2	K #7	SI #3		SI #4	K #7		
3	K #8	SI #3	K #7	SI #4	K #8		
4	K #8	SI #3	K #7	SI #4	K #8		
5	SP #4	SI #3	K #8	SI #4	SP #4		
6	SP #4	SI #3	K #8	SI #4	SP #4		

* While the days do not need to be exact, add the workouts *in this precise order* to your calendar.

Killer #7

Don't forget to warm up and cool down!
Take a 1 minute break in between each set.

Complete *3 sets of series one* and then *3 sets of series two.*

SERIES ONE

(COMPLETE 3 SETS OF FULL SERIES)

EXERCISE	REPS	WEIGHT
1 - Squat with V-Press	12 reps	Moderate Weight
2 - Plank Off Ball with Press-Outs	45 secs	Body Weight
3 - Ball Hamstring Curls	15 reps	Body Weight
4 - Side-to-Side Jump Lunges	15/side	Body Weight

SERIES TWO

(COMPLETE 3 SETS OF FULL SERIES)

EXERCISE	REPS	WEIGHT
1 - Side Plank with Top Leg Lift	8/side	Body Weight
2 - Burpees	10 reps	Body Weight
3 - Pushups Off Elevated Surface	8 reps	Body Weight
4 - Alternating Mid Row	12/side	Moderate Weight

Workout Complete!

Killer #8

Don't forget to warm up and cool down!
Take a 1 minute break in between each set.

Complete *3 sets of series one* and then *3 sets of series two*.

SERIES ONE

(COMPLETE 3 SETS OF FULL SERIES)

EXERCISE	REPS	WEIGHT
1 - Alternating Jump Lunges	10/side	Body Weight
2 - Single Arm and Leg Shoulder Press	12/side	Moderate Weight
3 - Single Leg Lunge with Weight	10/side	Light to Moderate Weight
4 - Spider Jump Pushups	8 reps	Body Weight

SERIES TWO

(COMPLETE 3 SETS OF FULL SERIES)

EXERCISE	REPS	WEIGHT
1 - Plank with Weight Slide	8/side	Light Weight
2 - Alternating Bench Press	12/side	Moderate Weight
3 - Lawnmower	12/side	Moderate Weight
4 - Side Plank with Arm Rotations	8/side	Body Weight

Workout Complete!

Super Pump #4

Don't forget to warm up and cool down!

Complete 2 sets of this series
with a 1 minute break in between each set.

EXERCISE	REPS	WEIGHT
1 - Alternating Jump Lunges	30 seconds	Body Weight
2 - Plank Off Ball with Press-Outs	30 seconds	Body Weight
3 - Side-to-Side Jump Lunges	30 seconds	Body Weight
4 - Pushups Off Toes, One Leg Elevated	30 seconds	Body Weight
5 - Alternating Bench Press	30 seconds	Moderate Weight
6 - Jumps with Foot Touches in the Air	30 seconds	Body Weight
7 - Ball Hamstring Curls	30 seconds	Body Weight

Workout Complete!

Sweaty Intervals #3

Don't forget to warm up and cool down!
Do as many reps of each exercise as you can in each round.
Each round consists of 30 seconds of exercise followed by a 30 second break.

Go as FAST as you can without compromising good technique.

EXERCISE	ROUNDS	WEIGHT
1 - Jacks	2	Body Weight
2 - High Knees	2	Body Weight
3 - Weighted Punches	2	Light Weight
4 - Wide Jump Squats/Low Jacks	3	Body Weight
5 - 180 Degree Squats	4	Body Weight
6 - Jumping Jack Planks	4	Body Weight

Workout Complete!

Sweaty Intervals #4

Don't forget to warm up and cool down!
Do as many reps of each exercise as you can in each round.
Each round consists of 30 seconds of exercise followed by a 30 second break.

Go as FAST as you can without compromising good technique.

EXERCISE	ROUNDS	WEIGHT
1 - Jacks	1	Body Weight
2 - High Knees	1	Body Weight
3 - Weighted Punches	1	Light Weight
4 - Wide Jump Squats/Low Jacks	2	Body Weight
5 - 180 Degree Squats	3	Body Weight
6 - Jumping Jack Planks	3	Body Weight
7 - Skier Over Yoga Mat	4	Body Weight
8 - Basketball Jumps	4	Body Weight

Workout Complete!

Well congratulations for making it this far. Cheers to you! Just imagine a cold one in your hand, and one in mine. But who are we kidding . . . we're using f*cking water, aren't we? But we feel pretty damn good, eh?

By the time I was "finished" the program, it had been a total of twenty-five weeks. Sure, there were a few slip-ups along the way, but it did not seem to affect my progress. Like Ang always said, if I was following the program 80% of the time, I would do fine!

Starting weight: 192 lbs.
Weight at 25 weeks in: 153 lbs.

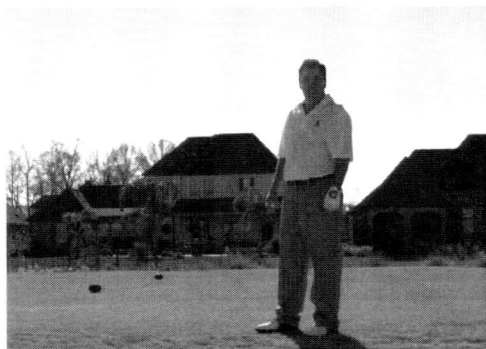

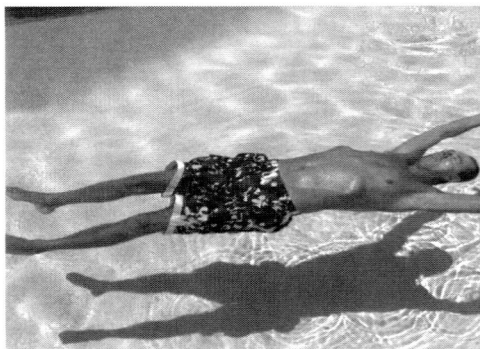

In the last weeks of this phase, Ang hopped across the border to visit us. I was proud of my accomplishments and knew I had done well, but it was the look on Ang's face when she saw me in person for the first time in six months that reinforced I had done a good job. I held myself together, but Ang cried her eyes out.

If you're entering the sustainability phase you might be feeling a little freaked out, like I was. Or maybe not. Either way, there are a few things to consider. Ang told me that upwards of 80% of people that lose weight will gain it all back (and often more) within a two year period. Why? Because it's really easy to get complacent! I don't understand it, but it seems to be the case for nearly everyone I talk to that has lost weight. We relax a bit with our portions, food choices, exercise routine, etc., and just like that we're back where we started.

I would have never guessed it, but I think maintaining a weight loss is even more effort than losing the weight in the first place.

Yeah, shit. It's because the weight loss is pretty fast in comparison to the rest of your life. That's right, the rest of your life. It's the piece most of us seem to forget. It's not about losing the weight and then being done and slowly going back to your old habits.

It's time to say goodbye to *Old You. New, Healthy You* is here to stay, but this requires you to keep up with the new habits you have worked so hard for.

I was feeling awesome about my results. I was back to my old fighting weight. I had so much energy, my flexibility improved for golf with the huge reduction in my gut, and I looked svelte! I wanted to get out and live life, so Diane and I went on a vacation we always dreamed of—a river cruise through Bordeaux, France. We spent two weeks drinking our favourite wine, indulging in spectacular French food, and sight seeing. In my mind we were walking a lot and the portions were small, so I would be fine to eat and drink whatever I wanted and would maintain my weight. It was fun . . . real fun! It was almost as if I was celebrating my achievement with a break in my new way of life.

But two weeks later I got home and stood on the scale to see a weight gain of 14 pounds! My pants were tight, my belly was slightly hanging over my belt again, and I felt ashamed. The shame turned to depression. I was so mad at myself for letting things go so far. To lose 14 pounds was going to take a lot of work. It was very clear to me how it could easily make a person so upset that they would just give in and go right back to their old ways.

I wish I could say it was no problem to jump right back into my new habits, but it wasn't. I was feeling deprived with the food choices, as they simply didn't compare to what I was eating on vacation. Getting back to my workouts was a little easier, but I could feel my stomach jiggle, and that made me feel crappy again. I had no choice. I printed off a habit tracker and started right from the beginning again.

Instead of going two weeks at a time with the habits, I chose to do every two days adding in the next habit. I focused on water then I slowly added each habit back in again. I didn't want to be a slave to the habit tracker for life, but it was clear I was not ready to wing it just yet. It took me a month to lose those 14 pounds! Two weeks to put it on, four weeks to take it off. It sucked.

I did learn, though, that weight gain will happen from time to time, be it due to complacency at home or a sweet vacation. It happens. But for me, I have committed to a threshold of five pounds. Any more than a five-pound weight gain and I find it mentally tough to get back into the groove. Depression sets in a bit and I really struggle. I don't like feeling this way, so I keep myself within these five pounds. I call it my wiggle room (pardon the pun). It's a reasonable amount of weight to think about losing. Anything more and it begins to feel daunting.

Any dip in my dedication leading to a weight gain nearing five pounds is a reminder that all of the old tendencies toward food and exercise are still there inside me. I've not gotten rid of them, I've just replaced them with new ones. It is just like smoking. I crave a cigarette every single day, but I choose to stick with my commitment. The same goes for my nutrition and exercise.

> Whenever I get onto that slippery slope situation, I pull out my habit tracker and post it back on the fridge to keep myself accountable.

I've had a lot of change in my life since the program. I finally retired from work, and Diane and I moved permanently to the US. I'm happy to say that during the move I did not miss a single workout. Our workout equipment was the last of our items to be packed and one of the first to be unpacked.

Once settled, I started to frequent our new neighbourhood's fitness centre. It was a one-mile jog away, so I used that as my warm-up. (I can't believe I just called that my warm-up . . . that used to be a daunting distance to run.) In the gym I would pull out my workout program and get right into it. As the weeks went on, I began to recognize faces of other gym-goers. People would look over at what I was doing every once in a while. I figured it was because I was grunting and sweating like a beast, but by this time I was no longer embarrassed about it; it was necessary to breathe properly and work at the intensity required of my workouts. Eventually those familiar faces began to approach me. I was getting questions about my training—about the specific exercises I was doing, the exercise sheet I brought with me, how many years I had been working out for, what I was training for, etc. I had no idea how much I had learned until I started talking with people at the gym who were in the position I was in just eight months prior. I started offering tips to people on how they could lose weight. Suddenly I was the "expert" in the gym! Get this: sometimes people who had never even spoken to me started copying my routines. For a very brief moment I questioned whether or not I was like the veiny guys in the '70s. Looking in the mirror brought me back to reality. For starters, my shorts were entirely too long to be those guys. But I was fit and feeling good, and thanks to my favourite daughter I certainly knew a lot more than most.

Reading and learning about fitness and nutrition will likely become a bit of a hobby now that you have come this far. It almost needs to be in order to keep the passion and momentum going. Have fun with it, but don't overthink it. You can confuse yourself and work yourself up trying to stay current with all the new research and exercise fads out there. It's okay to want to learn more and grow, but rely on your foundation of knowledge from this system and then use your common sense to decide if it is really worth trying.

When people start asking you for advice on exercises to do to lose weight (and believe me, they will) make sure you tell them that while working out is incredibly important, the key to the loss starts at nutrition. Heck, when they ask you for advice, tell them to go get this book!

TERRY'S TIPS

1. Give yourself some credit for what you just accomplished. This was NOT easy.... and you persevered and did it. That deserves some recognition.

2. You can easily talk yourself out of a workout, but you can also talk yourself back into it if you remind yourself of why this is important to you. Remind yourself of where you started. If you don't remember, keep an old photo of yourself on the fridge. I do, and it scares me away from cutting an extra hunk of cheese off the block, every time!

3. Two weeks completely off of your exercise program is too long . . . you will hurt when you go back! Make sure if you're taking a break that you're still doing your maintenance routines. You can maintain your weight with your nutrition, but you will not feel as healthy and strong if you don't have the exercise piece with it.

4. Do a quick check at every meal. To keep things really simple, every time you sit down to eat ask yourself this: Is half my plate veggies? Do I have a palm size of protein? Did I do a weight training workout? If

yes, do I have half a cup of carbohydrates? Is this perfect? No, but it is better than no awareness.

5. If you're feeling out of control or slipping a little, pull out a habit tracker as soon as possible. Write your workouts into your calendar so you don't miss them.

6. Give yourself permission to let loose every so often. There's something empowering about choosing to let loose in advance versus letting loose and having guilt or regret afterward.

7. So you had a bad day? A bad week? Ate a bit (or a lot) too much on holiday? Don't sweat it. Just get back on the wagon the next day . . . or better yet, at your next meal.

Whether at the gym, on the greens, or at a party with friends, it's rewarding to talk to people and share as much information as I can about my experiences with fitness and healthy eating (heck, that must be why I agreed to participate in this book!). Just as I used to be, people are often skeptical about my methods and results. They think I'm just not eating very much anymore or spending hours and hours on a treadmill everyday. They want tips and tricks they can implement for instant results. I definitely sound more and more like Ang when talking to people like that, because I know that quick solutions are never an answer. It's more complicated. In order to make it happen you have to be fully open to changing many (or in my case, most) of your tendencies. It requires an overwhelming desire to change, a clear focus, persistence, and consistency along with a plan like the one Ang has laid out here. I'm reluctant to call this the end of the program. While it is the end of this book, in life it is not . . . you're just getting started.

EPILOGUE

It's been nearly five years since I put pen to paper and began writing this book. As in every industry, things change. New studies are released, new ideas are developed, and new fads are created. As the years roll on, three prevalent elements to every successful weight loss program remain.

1. Eating natural/less processed foods as often as possible.
2. Tracking/maintaining an awareness about what you are eating.
3. Keeping a consistent effort for short term and long term success.

With these three elements in mind, I created this program for my favourite dad with the intention of selecting sound nutrition habits that would create a systemized and track-able routine for him to follow, slowly introducing natural foods every couple of weeks in the most stress-free way I could think of to keep him engaged in this "healthy shit."

Reality Fitness has stood the test of time.

My dad has successfully kept the weight off all these years. Sure, he fluctuates from time to time when he has been on vacation and has had a few extra cellies. Every once in a while even at home he'll catch himself falling into old habits . . . skipping breakfast from time to time, having a larger portion than recommended, or missing workouts. It's his threshold weight gain of five pounds that motivates him to reel himself back in. After years of practicing being in tune with his body, he begins to feel off and goes back to the foundational habits he built. My dad now understands there is nothing wrong with adding in new elements. He finds himself intrigued with new fitness gadgets, foods, and trends, but he always stays true to the foundation. As long as you have a solid base to begin with—one that you can lean back on if the fad is not working for you—you'll always feel and be in control.

As my dad ages, he is finding his body is more susceptible to injury and his posture needs improvement, so his workout program has shifted from muscular endurance training and cardiovascular workouts to more strength and muscle building workouts. He still does not enjoy it, but he clearly understands the value since he continues to keep at it! He finally realizes that you are never done. A routine might evolve over time, but the foundation is always there and you can always build on it.

> A fitness and nutrition program is one you have for life, not six weeks, three months, or even six months.

Reading through this book again is a trip down memory lane. When I think about what my dad accomplished, the steady changes he made, the vulnerability, and the trust he put in me, it brings tears to my eyes. He's endured and conquered a lot of discomfort through dietary changes and a few sets of lunges. :) He made a promise to himself to get healthy, and he has stuck with it. His dedication, resiliency, and work ethic are just a few of his qualities I admire so much. It is so empowering to follow through with what you say you are going to do, and I can't think of anything more inspiring to others. My favourite dad continues to inspire me every day. I feel honoured to have been a part of his achievement, and grateful he allowed me to share his story in an effort to help others.

I remember the day when my dad first mentioned participating in an organized running race. He had been incrementally building up his running distances and reporting back with a play by play on his progress every few weeks. It was really cool to see how he used the same format we had used with his nutrition and applied it to his running. I was ecstatic about the idea of my favourite dad training and competing in an organized running event. In an effort to not scare him off, I played it cool and let the idea marinate a bit in his mind as he built his confidence to enter. I was 100% sure of his ability to run it, and to run it well, but he needed to feel the same way too.

Running was always a part of Ang's life. I used to stand on the side of the road during her marathons and watch her run by. To me, it was impressive (but also kind of crazy) to run for that long. After each run, Ang would get a T-shirt with the race name and sponsors on it, and she would give it to me because I thought they were neat. Never did I think I would be training for one of these races too.

You've already read how running seemed to just creep into my fitness life somehow over the course of the program. The more I incorporated running into the completion of my 10,000 steps, the more I began to enjoy it. In the beginning I would start by running for thirty seconds and then walking for two minutes to get my breath back. Then I progressed to one minute of running without stopping and two minutes of walking to catch my breath. Every time I went out for my walk to complete my 10,000 steps I would challenge myself to run just a little bit longer each time, even if it was just thirty seconds more. Eventually I began to notice my endurance improving. When I was able to run for thirty minutes straight, I began to increase my speed just a little bit every time. I eventually nudged myself to a level of fitness that gave me the confidence to casually bring up the idea with Ang about participating in a five kilometre race. Of course she was all over it. A few weeks later she sent me a text with dates for the Edmonton Father's Day Run—a five kilometre race that would support the Heart and Stroke Foundation. And just like that, the decision was made and the idea became much more real. Amazing! Less than a year before, I was barely able to run for more than twenty seconds at a time. TWENTY SECONDS. Now I was planning on participating in an organized run. Anybody that would have known me as the chain-smoking, coffee slugging workaholic would not believe it. Heck, I am still in disbelief myself!

At this point I was maintaining my Reality Fitness habits and running about 2.5 kilometres regularly, but I still had a bit of preparation to do before the event. Every day I focused on going just a little bit further than I had the day before. I did not worry too much about my speed, just the distance. Once I was able to complete the distance without a break, then I worked on going a bit faster. Ang insisted that just doing the race was a big enough accomplishment, but I didn't think so. My plan was to complete the run in less than thirty minutes.

I arrived in Edmonton a few days before the Father's Day run so I could play a few rounds of golf and have a few beers with the boys. It was a good time, but I had the race in the back of my mind. I was starting to worry. What if I couldn't go as fast as I had planned?

The day of the race we drove downtown and found our place in line to cross the starting point. Ang had her watch on and was in charge of keeping track of the time while we ran the length of the route together. I was in charge of setting the pace—this was my race to conquer. My heart was pounding before we even started running, and I felt like I needed to pee like a racehorse. All of sudden the bell rang and we were off!

The first part of the course was all down hill. That was nice to build up a bit of speed, but I realized that we would have that hill on the way back too. It was probably the adrenaline and a bit of nervousness that led me to run quite a bit faster than my planned race pace. By the time we reached the halfway point, I was dying. Normally I didn't feel like I needed water during my runs until afterward, but I grabbed a cup from one of the volunteers at the first opportunity. It brought me back to the workouts when I "needed to fill my water bottle up." I wanted to be anywhere but there. My lungs and my legs hurt so badly. Somehow, though, I kept moving. I told myself that stopping was not an option. When Ang gave me my time just after the halfway mark it gave me a glimmer of hope. I was ahead of schedule! I pushed on with Ang encouraging me along the way.

> I couldn't talk.
> All my energy had to go into running and not puking.

We eventually made it to the final hill that led to the finish line. It was a curvy hill with switchbacks. We made it through the first turn, but then I had to stop. All I could say was: "Sorry. Sorry. Sorry." Ang would later tell me that we had stopped for only about fifteen seconds. Just that very brief moment of relief was all I needed to muster up the energy to get to the top, though. I'm not sure how it helped, but it did. My legs felt like I was running through waist deep water, but they were still moving. The finish line was in sight, and the running lane was lined with cheering volunteers and supportive family members. I sprinted as quickly as I could under the finish banner, and Ang clicked her watch off to set my final time. I was scared to ask.

28:11.

I did it! I was so relieved and so satisfied with the result. It was another accomplishment I had never imagined in my future, even just months ago.

I put my first official race T-shirt on; that I had earned for myself, and delightfully discovered it was too big!

After quitting smoking, choosing to commit to the Reality Fitness program has been the best decision I have made for my health and for my future. The incremental steps, week after week, leading to my fitness and weight transformation have changed my life.

Not only did it improve my health, but I have also applied the process of this system to other areas of my life.

I learned that there is a lot less frustration when you are not trying to change everything all at once. The experience of seeing how one manageable change at a time can lead to really big results has helped me accomplish new feats that I otherwise might have been too intimidated or overwhelmed to even attempt.

I'm not the type to hype myself up or boast about my accomplishments, but this is an exception. I have maintained my weight loss and now focus on staying healthy and fit so I can enjoy my retirement for years to come. I continue to run and incorporate fitness into my life, through a variety of activities, on a consistent basis. It is easier now that I have more time with retirement, but the desire and effort still have to be there to be successful, and with my favourite daughter by my side, I can't go wrong.

THANK YOU

To embrace the *Reality Fitness* program requires patience, a true desire to change, a positive attitude, and the willingness to be honest with yourself about your habits. I thank you so much for picking up this book, taking time out of your life to read it, and for trusting in the process enough to apply the advice.

Whether you have reached that point where you feel good in your skin, or you are still in the process of getting there, continue to be in tune with your body. Use successful completion of the habits as success markers, not just your weight, and remind yourself as often as you can that you are actively doing something positive to better your health and your life.

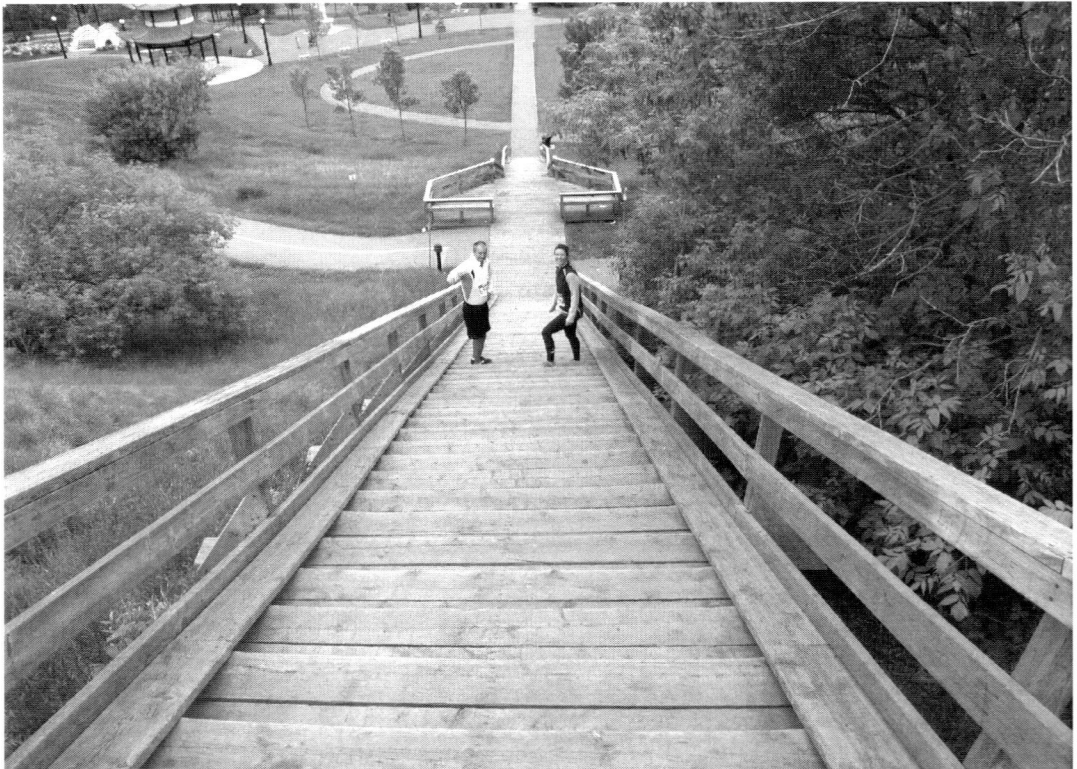

REALITY FITNESS
APPENDICES

APPENDIX A: WARM-UPS

There are two different warm-ups provided in this program. The first warm-up uses a foam roller to massage your muscles, allowing for increased blood flow to the tighter areas of your body. Time permitting, use the foam roller on each area of your body for 30 seconds each. For areas of your body that are tighter, use a bit more time if necessary. If you are shorter on time, at the very least focus on rolling out your tightest muscles for 30 seconds each, then proceed to the second warm-up.

The second warm-up provided is a dynamic warm-up, which helps your body transition from a cold, static state to a warm, mobile state while gently raising your heart rate. Dynamic movements help improve functional range of motion through the joints, and they increase blood supply to the muscles to prime your body for the workout you are about to embark on!

PDF downloads of the warm-ups to print or to pull up on
your favourite device are available at:
www.realityfitnessbook.com

QUADRICEPS (FRONT OF LEG)

Foam Roller Warm-up

Lie down with the front of your thighs on top of the foam roller. Use your hands to slowly push yourself forward and back over the roller between your hip and knee joints. For a more intense pressure, lift one leg up or rest it on top of the other leg.

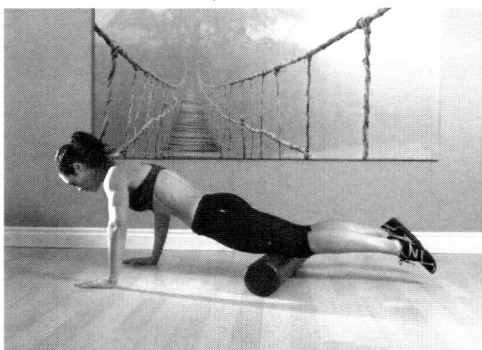

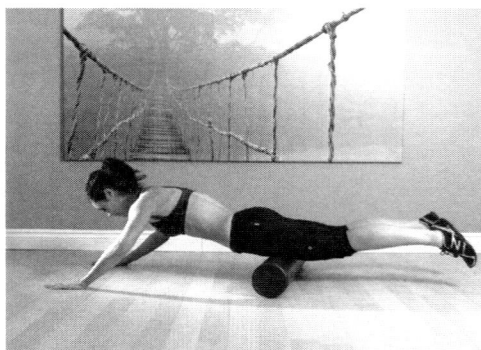

GLUTES (BUTTOCKS)
Foam Roller Warm-up

Seated squarely on the foam roller, lean to one side until only one side of your buttock is in contact with the roller. With your hands behind you, and your feet placed on the floor, slowly roll the side of your buttock back and forth by using a push/pull motion with your hands and feet. Repeat on the other side.

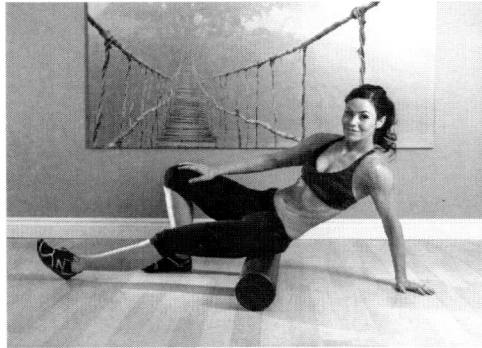

ILIOTIBIAL BAND (SIDE OF LEG & HIP)

Foam Roller Warm-up

Seated on the foam roller, lean to one side until the side of your leg (below the hip joint) is in contact with the roller. With your hand behind you, and your foot placed on the floor in front of the leg that is being rolled out, slowly roll the side of your hip and leg (the IT band) back and forth using a push/pull motion with your hand and foot.

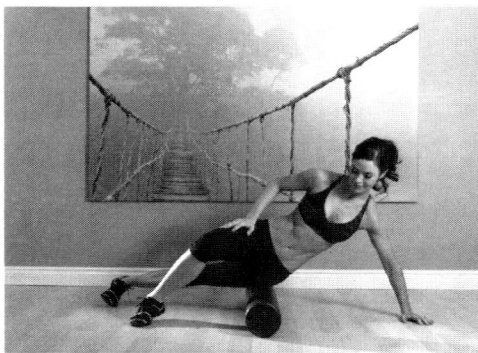

GASTROCNEMIUS & SOLEUS (CALF MUSCLES)
Foam Roller Warm-up

Rest the backs of your lower legs on the foam roller. Lift your body up with your hands behind you and slowly push and pull your legs (between the ankle and knee joints) with your hands. For more intense pressure, cross your legs so only one leg is resting on the foam roller at a time.

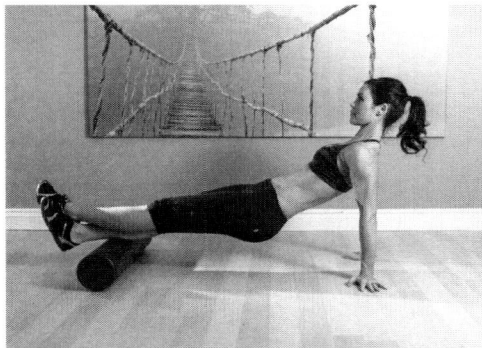

If you are unable to lift your body weight up in this position, lie flat on your stomach and have someone roll the foam roller over the back of your lower legs as if using a rolling pin.

LATISSIMUS DORSI (BACK MUSCLES, UNDERNEATH THE ARMPIT)

Foam Roller Warm-up

Lie on your side with one arm up and over the foam roller. The point of contact should be the area of your rib cage just beneath your armpit. Just holding here might be enough pressure as is. If you want more pressure, place one foot in front of you and use that to slowly push and pull your body weight over the foam roller, going no further than ½ a roll of the foam roller.

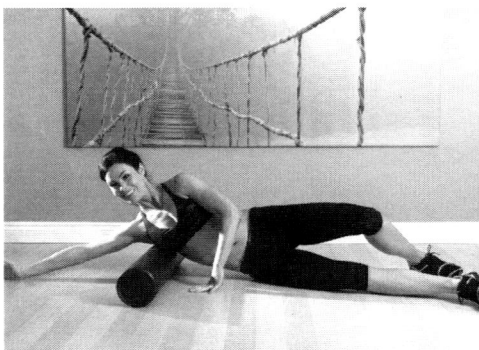

DELTOIDS & LATISSIMUS DORSI
(SHOULDER & BACK MUSCLES)
Foam Roller Warm-up

Begin by kneeling on the ground. Place your wrists on a foam roller two feet in front of you. Slowly roll the foam roller (using your wrists) away from your hips and press your chest toward the ground. You should feel this stretch in your lats and the front of your shoulders. Hold this position for 30 seconds, and then gently roll in the reverse direction out of the posture.

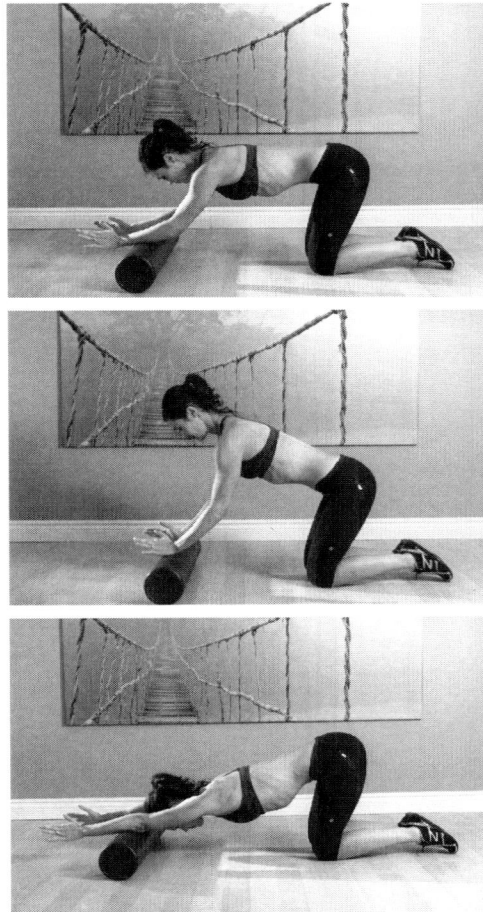

ARM ROLLS

Dynamic Warm-up
Length of time: 1 minute for each arm

In a standing position, swing one arm at a time in a forward direction for 30 seconds. Stop and switch, swinging in a backward direction for 30 seconds.

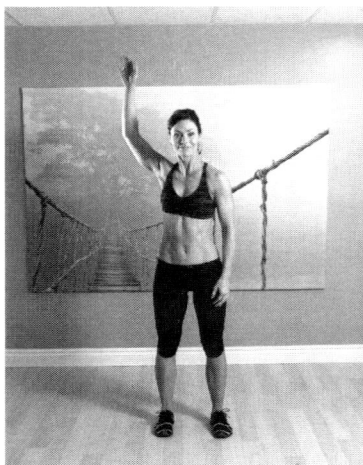

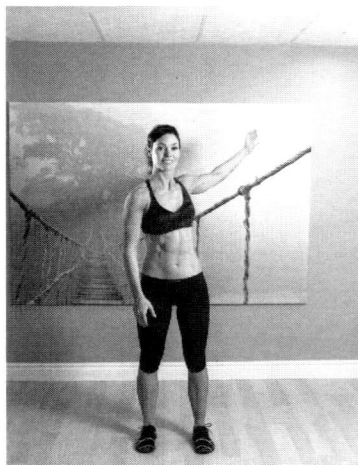

HIP ROTATIONS

Dynamic Warm-up
Length of time: 30 seconds per leg

In a standing position, raise one leg up to a 90-degree angle, bent at the knee. Rotate your leg in a circular motion as far out as your hips will allow and then back to the front without letting your foot touch the ground between rotations. Do not let your balancing knee twist while you rotate the other leg, and keep the balancing knee slightly bent.

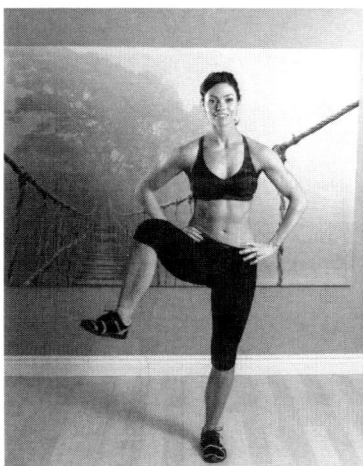

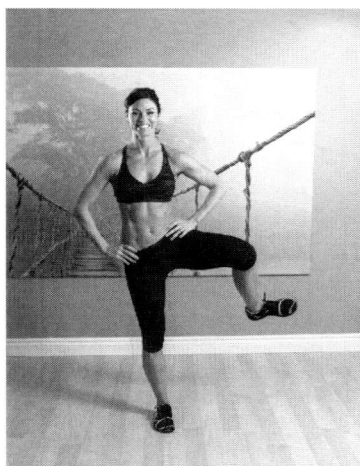

WALKOUTS

Dynamic Warm-up
Length of time: 1 minute

Start in a standing position. Bend at the waist and place your hands on the floor (if necessary, bend your knees slightly). Once your hands are on the floor, slowly walk one hand out at time until your back is parallel to the floor (a plank position with your hands located directly under your shoulders). Pause, then walk one hand at a time back toward your feet. Once you reach your feet, stand back up.

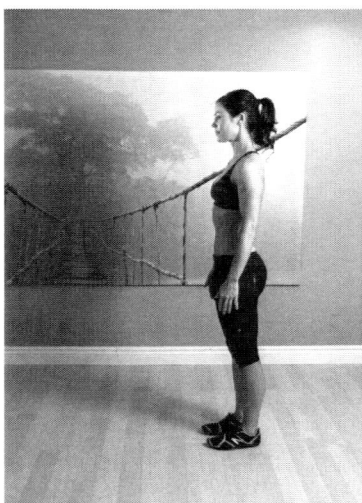

Start and end each walkout standing up.

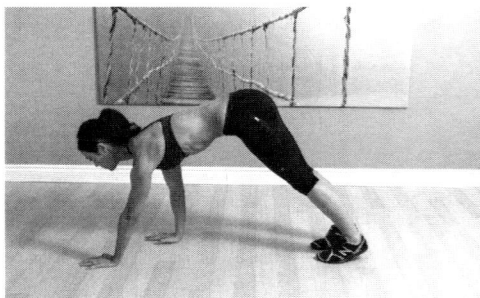

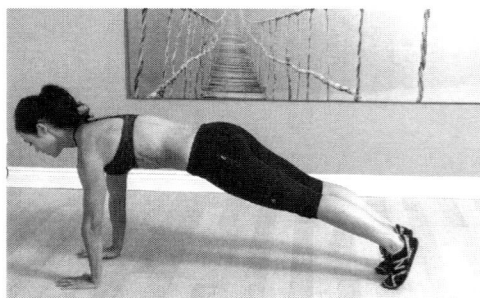

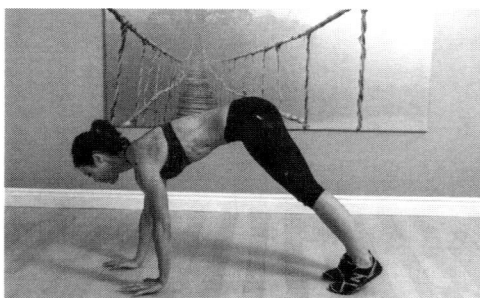

DEEP SUMO SQUATS

Dynamic Warm-up
Length of time: 1 minute

Stand with your feet a few inches wider than shoulder-width apart, with your toes pointing slightly outwards. Bend at the knees, then the hips, and squat down as low as you can go. If you have knee pain, do not go beyond 90 degrees. Be sure to keep your hips back far enough so that your knees stay overtop of your ankles. Pause, then move your chest forward while lengthening your legs at the same time (you will be in a floppy bent over position). Slowly curl yourself up to a standing position.

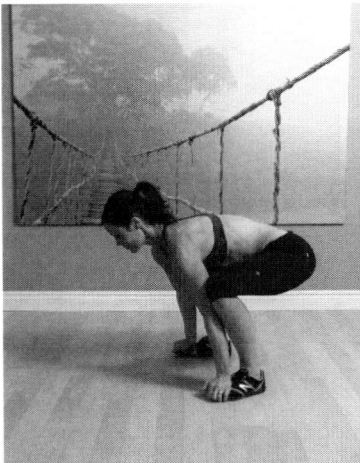

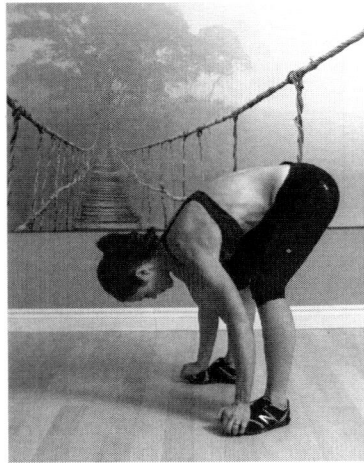

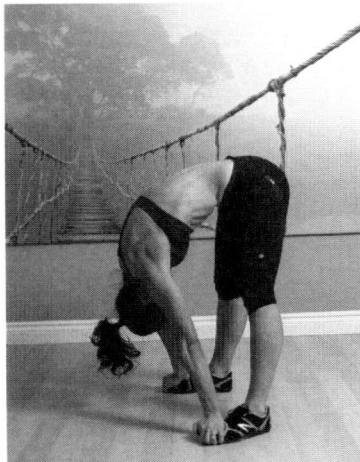

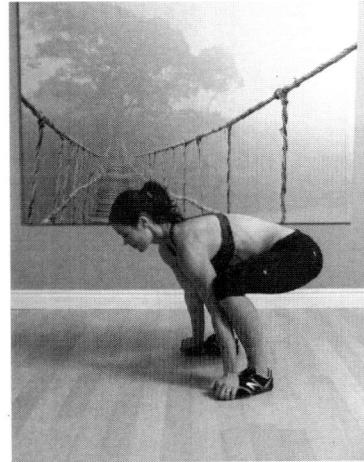

FOUR CORNER HOPS

Dynamic Warm-up
Length of time: 30 seconds per leg

Stand on one foot and jump about one ruler length between four imaginary corners of a box. Repeat this for 30 seconds per leg.

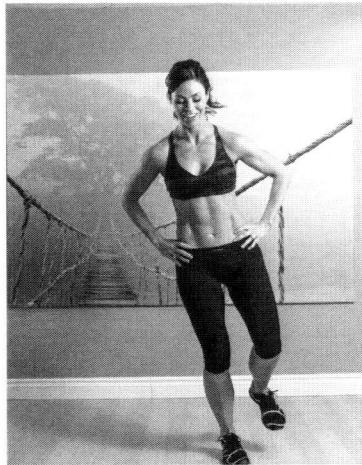

LONG JUMPS

Dynamic Warm-up
Length of time: 1 minute

Stand with your feet shoulder-width apart. Bend at the knees and the hips, and swing your arms as far back as you can. Use your momentum to take a giant leap/jump forward. Try to land on the heels of your feet.

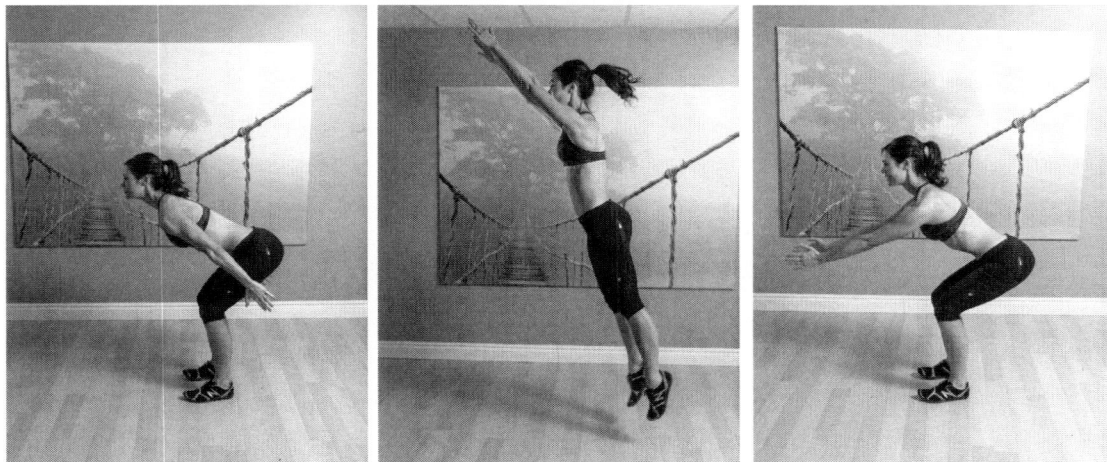

APPENDIX B: THE EXERCISES

Revisit the section on proper technique and breathing prior to starting your workout (pages 57-59).

Unless otherwise specified, each description explains the process for a single repetition of the exercise.

PDF downloads of the workouts to print or to pull up on your favourite device are available at: www.realityfitnessbook.com

180 DEGREE SQUATS

Appears in: Sweaty Intervals #3, #4
Targeted Muscles: Front, back & inner legs; Buttocks; Calves; Your heart!

Starting in a squat position (see Base Squat to review), jump and turn your body around in the air. Catch yourself in another squat 180 degrees from your starting position. Continue with this movement as quickly as possible, rotating in the same direction for the specified amount of time or repetitions. Repeat in the opposite direction.

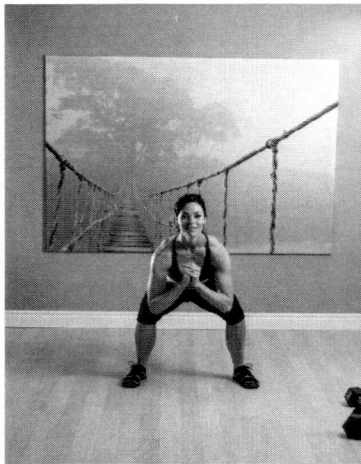

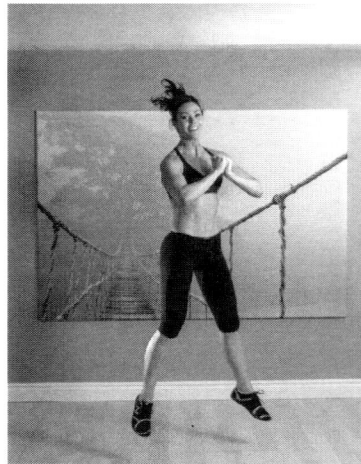

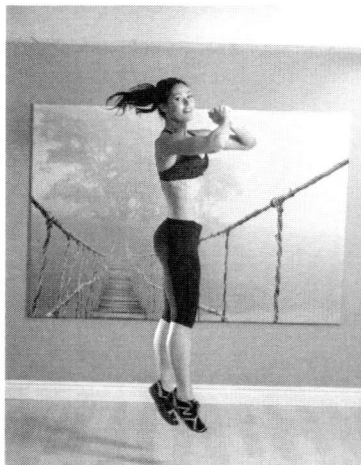

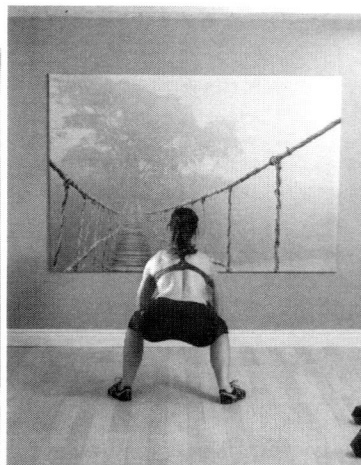

ALTERNATING BACK LUNGE

Appears in: Killer #1
Targeted Muscles: Front & back of legs; Buttocks

Take a large step back and bend both of your knees to 90 degrees so that your back knee almost touches the floor. Keep your front knee tracking with your ankle. Push through your front heel and stand up, placing both feet back together. Repeat, moving back with the opposite leg.

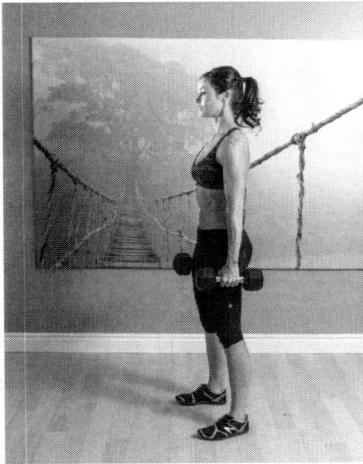

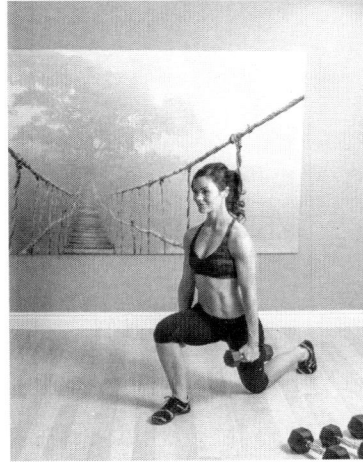

ALTERNATING BENCH PRESS (PHOTOS ON NEXT PAGE)

Appears in: Killer #8, Super Pump #4
Targeted Muscles: Front & backs of arms; Shoulders; Chest

With a dumbbell in each hand, lie on your back with your knees bent and feet flat on the floor. Start with arms extended, both weights above your chest. Slowly lower one arm at a time maintaining a 90-degree angle in your arm (your wrist should track over your elbow as you lower the weight down). Lower your arm down as far as possible without resting your elbow on the floor. Pause at the bottom for one second, then press the weight back up to the starting position. Perform the same movement with the other arm.

ALTERNATING BENCH PRESS (CONTINUED)

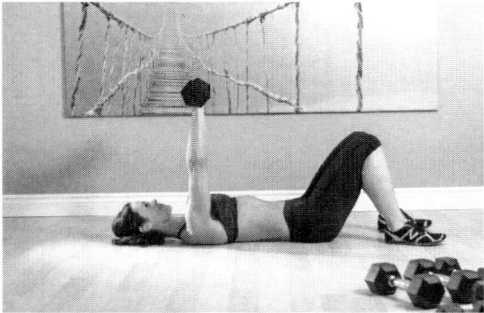

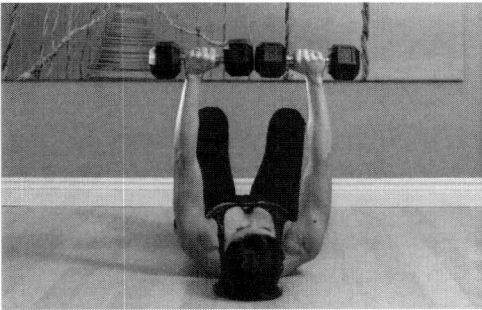

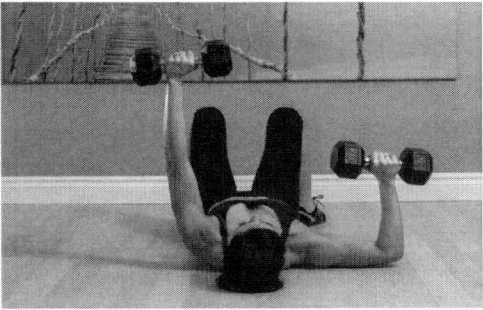

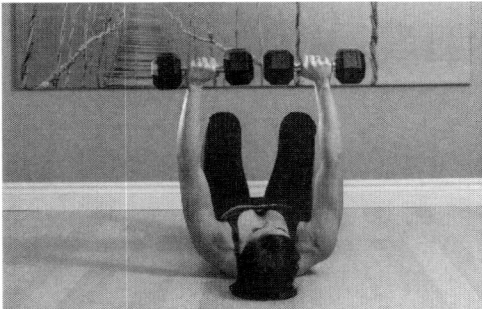

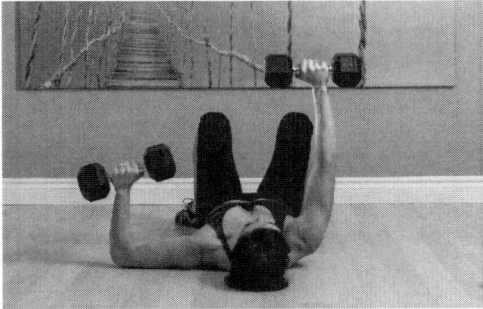

ALTERNATING JUMP LUNGES

Appears in: Killer #8, Super Pump #4
Targeted Muscles: Front & back of legs; Buttocks; Abdominals

Start from standing with your hands on your hips and take one large step forward bending both your knees at 90 degrees to form a lunge. From this position, jump vertically and while in the air switch your legs to land back down in another lunge with the opposite leg position. Each jump is considered one repetition.

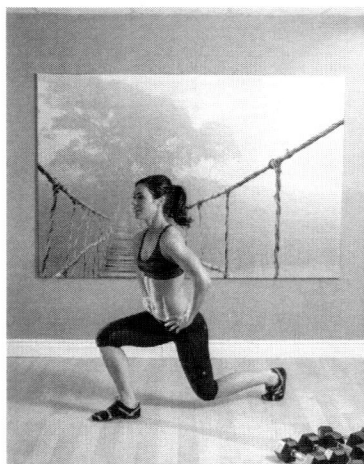

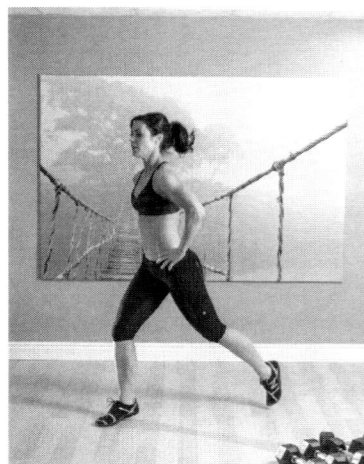

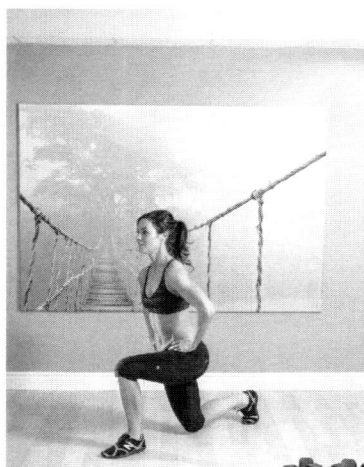

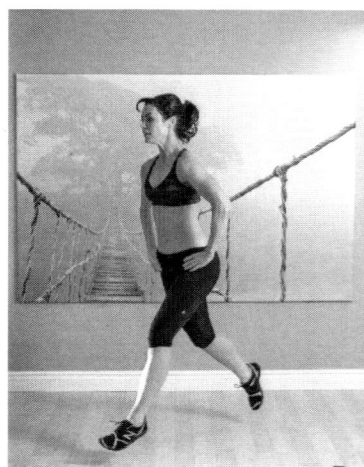

ALTERNATING MID ROW

Appears in: Killer #4, #7
Targeted Muscles: Upper back; Front & back of arms; Shoulders; Abdominals

Stand with your feet shoulder-width apart. Bend your knees slightly and flex your torso forward, keeping your back flat. Squeeze your buttocks to maintain a strong core, and keep your weight in your heels. Slowly bring one weight up and down at a time (alternating) toward your rib cage.

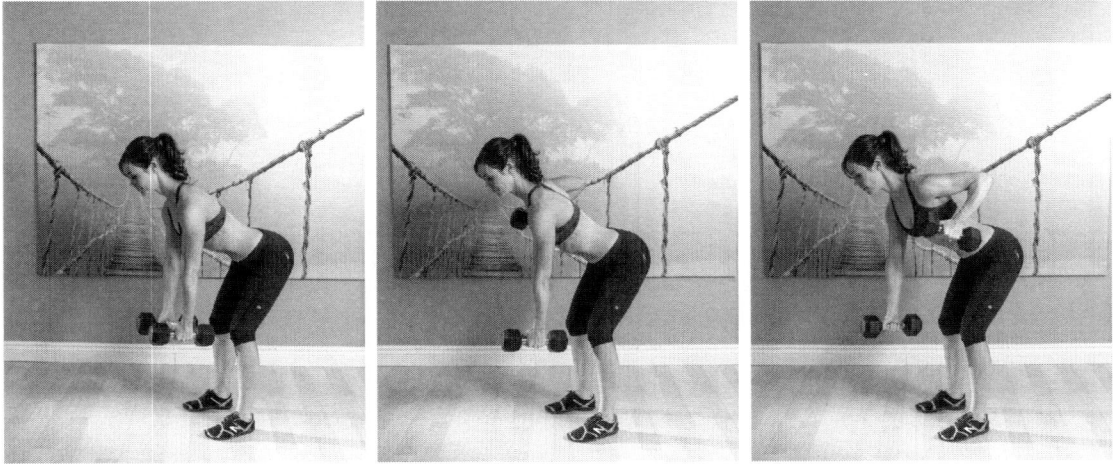

BACK LUNGE WITH FORWARD KICK

Appears in: Killer #4, Super Pump #2
Targeted Muscles: Front & back of legs; Calves; Buttocks

With or without weights in your hands (depending on your fitness level), take a large step backward into a lunge. Your back knee should be just an inch off the floor and your front knee should track nicely over the top of your ankle. Stand back up out of the lunge by pushing through your front heel. Swing your back leg forward into a kick and then step back into the lunge. Challenge your balance by not touching the ground during this transition. Complete the specified repetitions with one leg, and then repeat with the other leg.

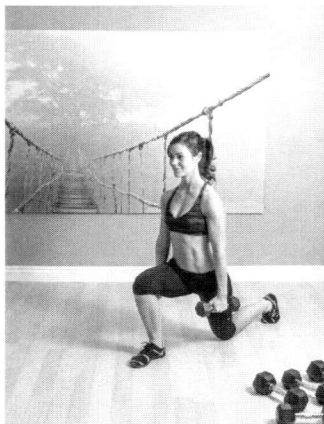

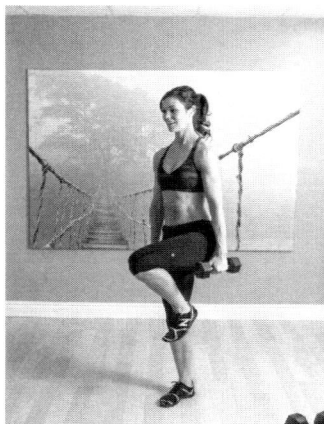

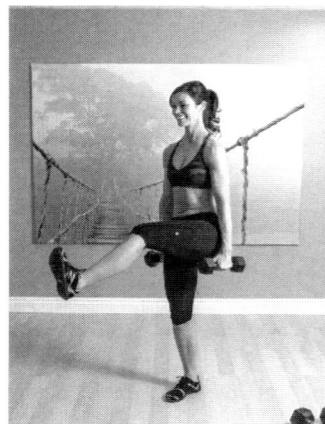

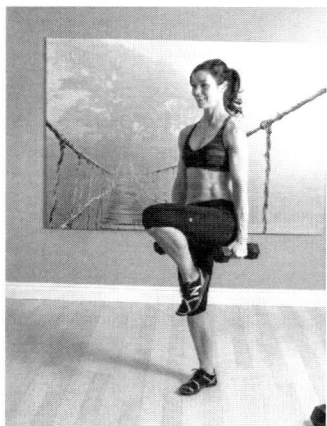

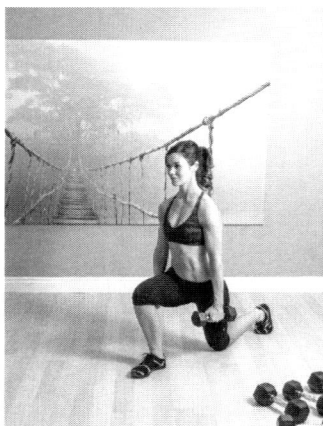

BALL HAMSTRING CURLS

Appears in: Killer #7, Super Pump #4
Targeted Muscles: Back of legs; Calves; Buttocks; Abdominals

Lie on your back and place your heels top and centre on your exercise ball. Flex your feet (point your toes to the ceiling), and elevate your hips off the floor. Avoid arching your back by engaging your abdominal and buttock muscles. Once in this position, slowly push your heels into the ball and drag it inward to your buttocks. Pause, then push the ball out with your feet, keeping your hips up the entire time.

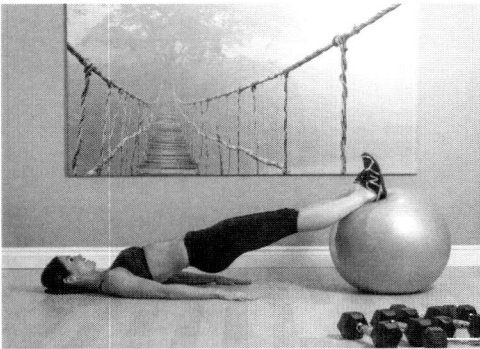

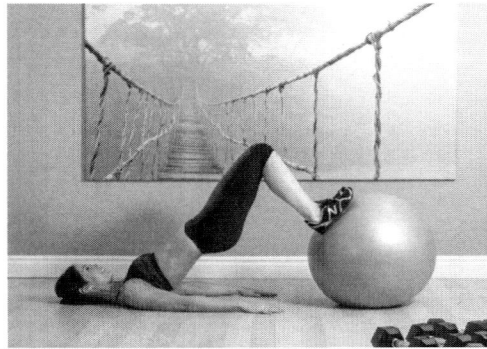

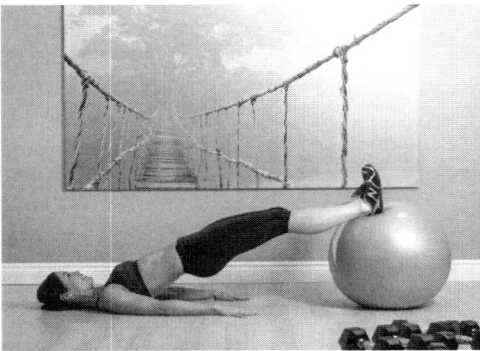

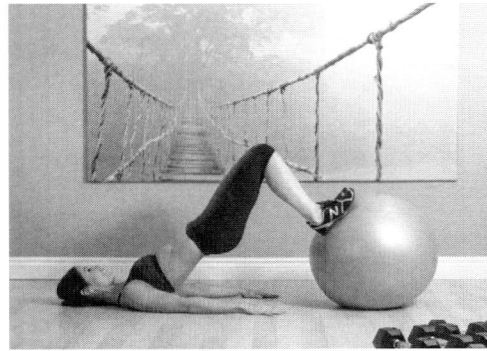

BALL PASS (PHOTOS ON NEXT PAGE)

Appears in: Killer #5
Targeted Muscles: Abdominals

Lie down on your back with an exercise ball in your hands. Lift your feet and arms upward simultaneously until they meet in the middle. Pass the ball from between your hands to between your feet and then lower your feet (with the ball) and your arms back down to just one inch off the floor (avoid touching the ground). Complete the specified repetitions, counting a single rep as passing the ball from your feet to your hands and then hands to your feet.

BALL PASS (CONTINUED)

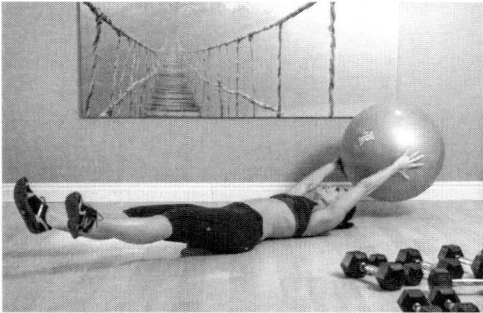

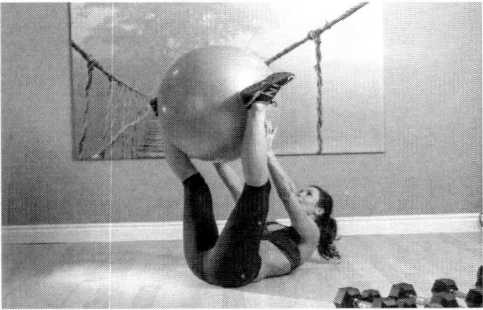

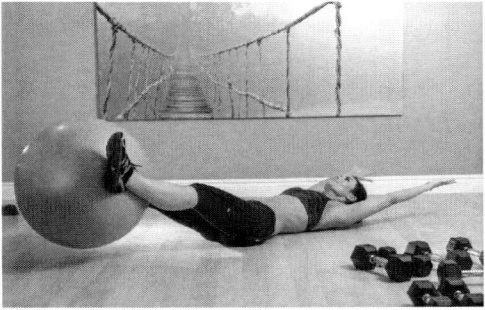

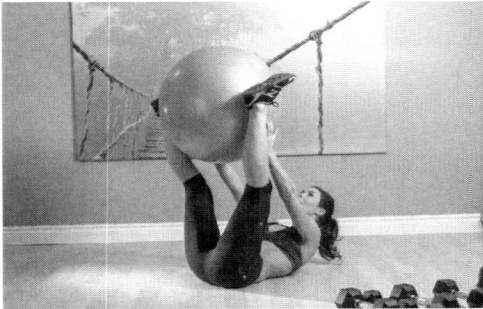

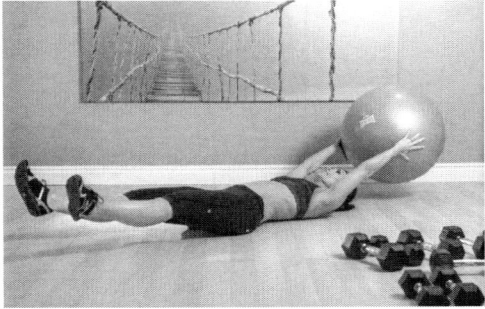

BASE PLANK (OFF ELBOWS OR HANDS)

Targeted Muscles: Abdominals; Shoulders

Lying on your stomach, place your forearms and hands on the floor with your elbows directly under your shoulders. Lift your body up off the floor using the pressure from your arms and your toes. Tilt your tailbone toward the floor (as if you were slightly tucking your buttocks underneath you). This helps to isolate your abdominal muscles. Hold this position for the specified amount of time.

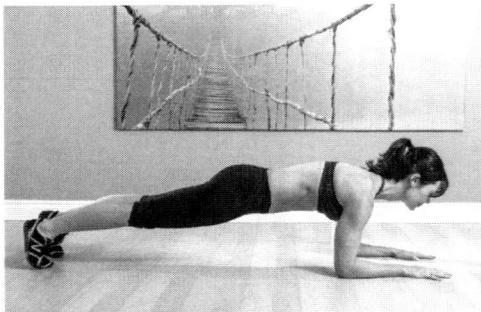

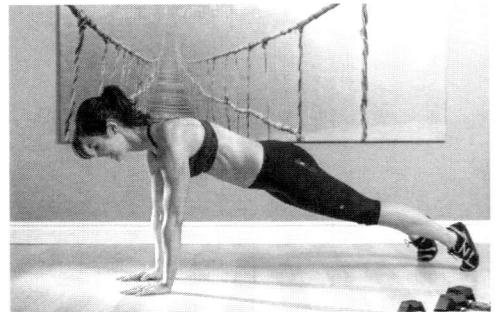

BASE SQUAT

Targeted Muscles: Front & back of legs; Buttocks

Stand with your feet shoulder-width apart (the inside of your foot should be in line with the outside of your shoulder). Bend at your hips and knees to lower into a squat position (as if you're about to sit in a chair) until your thighs are just past parallel to the floor. If you have knee problems, do not go past parallel. Keep your knees over top of your ankles (you should be able to see your toes throughout the entire movement). Maintain good posture by keeping your chest up as high as you can as you lower into the squat and while you stand back up to complete each repetition.

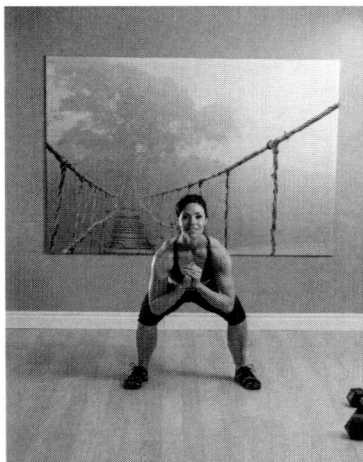

BASKETBALL JUMPS

Appears in: Sweaty Intervals #4
Targeted Muscles: Front, back & inner legs; Buttocks; Calves; Your heart!

Starting in a squat position (see Base Squat to review), jump and lift your arms up as if you are making a basketball jump shot. Land back into a squat and repeat the jumping movement as quickly as you can for the specified amount of time.

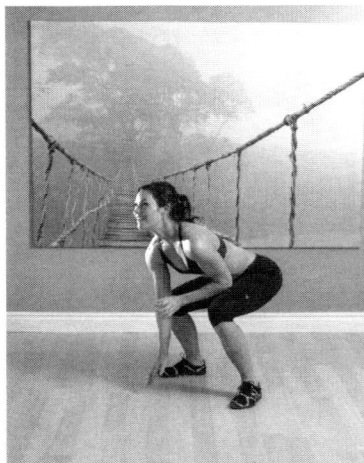

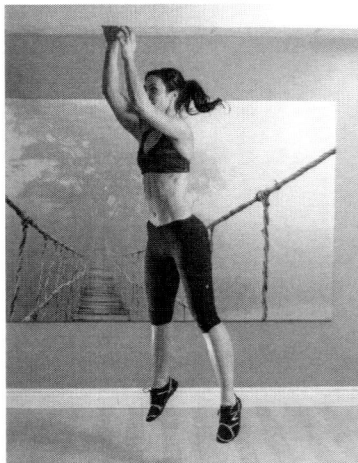

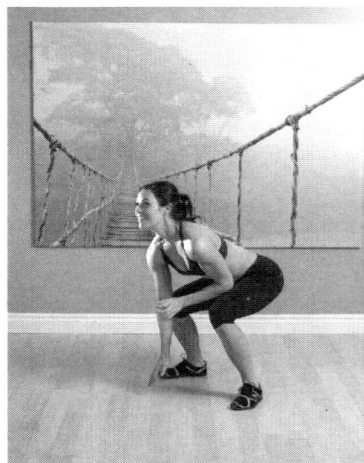

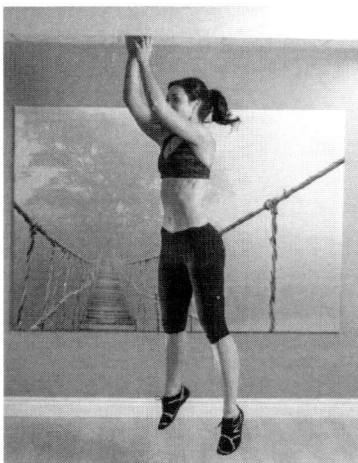

BENCH PRESS OFF FLOOR

Appears in: Killer #2
Targeted Muscles: Front & back of arms; Shoulders; Chest

With a dumbbell in each hand, lie on your back with your knees bent and feet flat on the floor. Start with both weights above your chest and your arms extended. Slowly and simultaneously lower both weights down to your sides to a 90-degree angle in your arms (your wrists should track over your elbows as you lower the weights). Lower your arms down as far as possible without resting your elbows on the floor. Pause at the bottom for one second, then press the weights back up to the starting position.

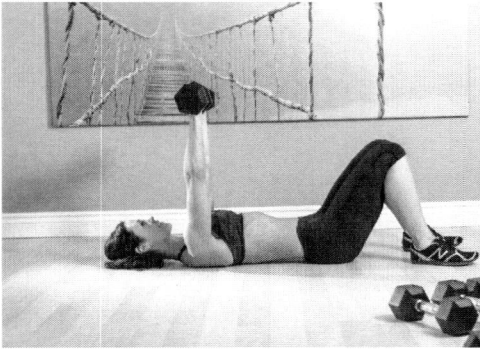

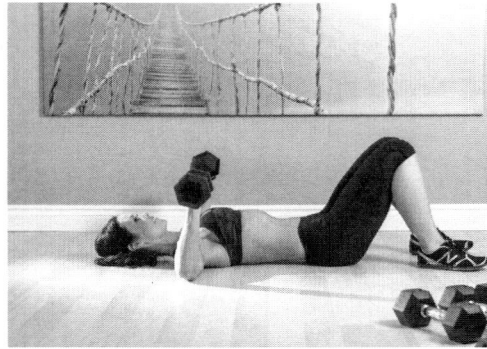

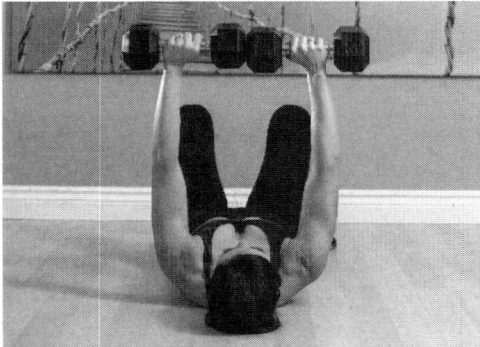

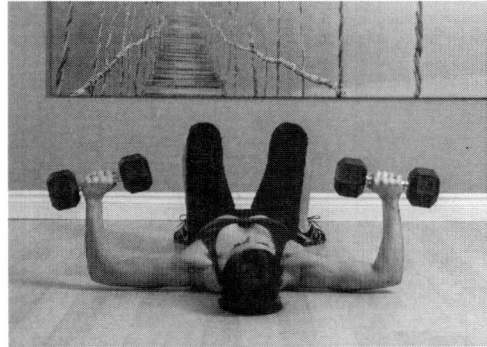

BILATERAL MID ROW

Appears in: Killer #2, Super Pump #1
Targeted Muscles: Upper back; Front & back of arms; Shoulders; Abdominals

Holding a weight in each hand (palms facing toward each other), stand with your feet shoulder-width apart. Bend slightly at your hips and knees, and flex your torso forward while you maintain a flat back. Squeeze your buttocks to maintain a strong core, and keep your weight in your heels. Slowly bring both weights up toward your rib cage and then slowly lower them back down.

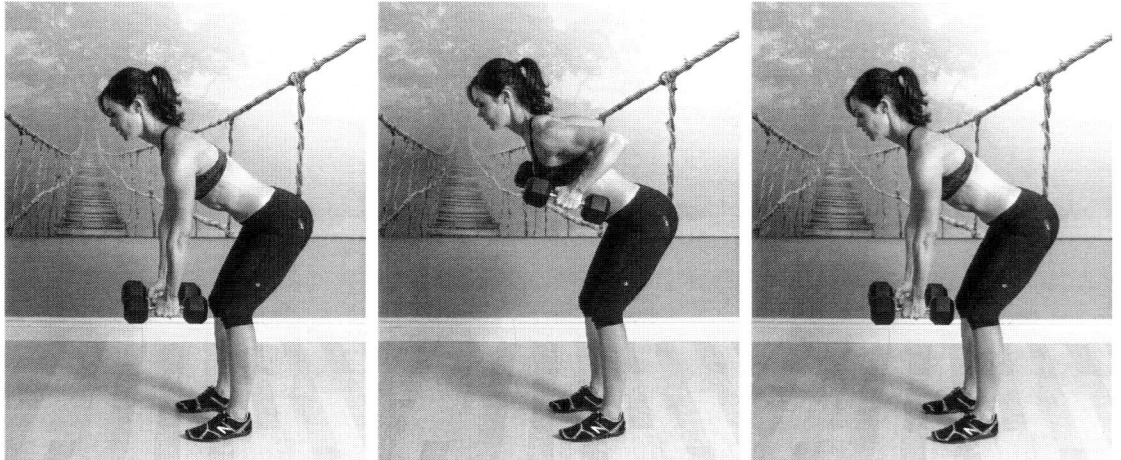

BURPEES

Appears in: Killer #7

Targeted Muscles: Front & back of legs; Upper back; Shoulders; Abdominals; Chest; Your heart!

Place your hands on the floor, jump both of your feet back simultaneously into a plank position, then jump both feet back up simultaneously to a kneeling position. Stand up and jump. This is one repetition.

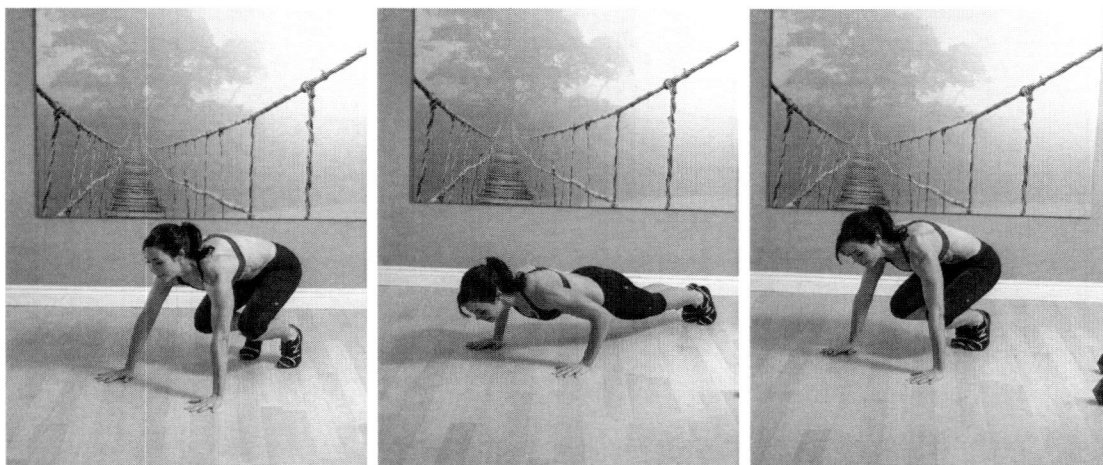

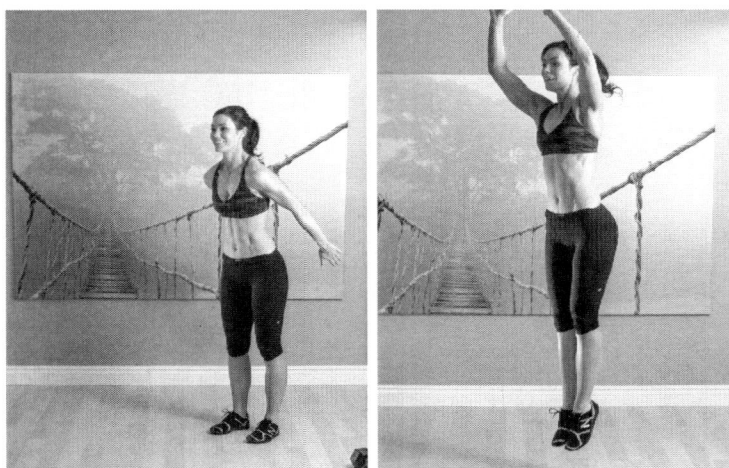

FROG PLANKS (PHOTOS ON NEXT PAGE)

Appears in: Killer #5
Targeted Muscles: Shoulders; Abdominals; Front & back of arms; Upper back

Start in a plank position up on your toes and with your hands directly underneath your shoulders. With a tight core (tilt your tailbone toward the floor), slowly lower your body down onto your right forearm and then onto your left forearm. Push back up with your right hand first and then onto your left hand. When pushing yourself up, be sure to place your hand directly under your shoulder to isolate the muscles and protect the shoulder joint. Repeat this process initiating the lowering and raising with the right arm. Complete the specified number of repetitions and then switch, leading with the left arm for the next round.

FROG PLANKS (CONTINUED)

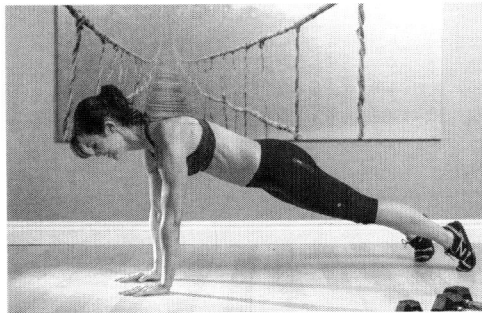

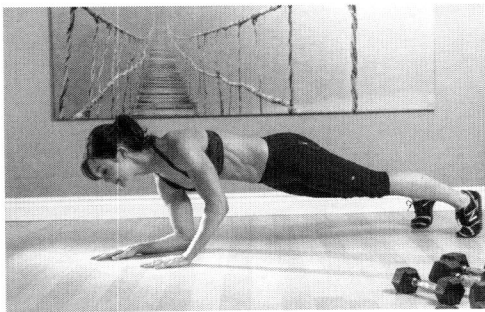

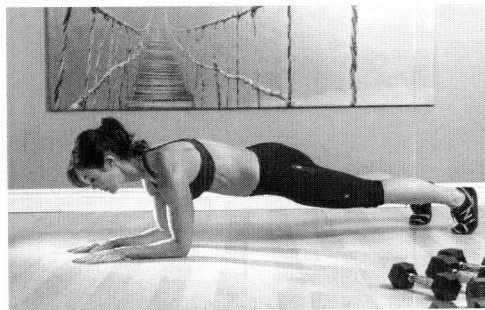

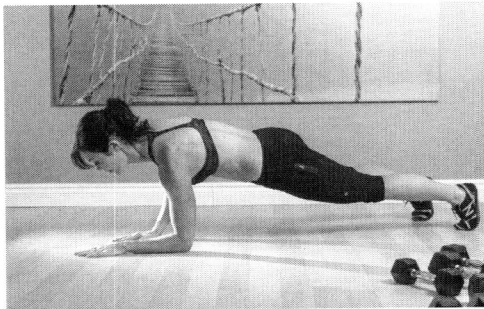

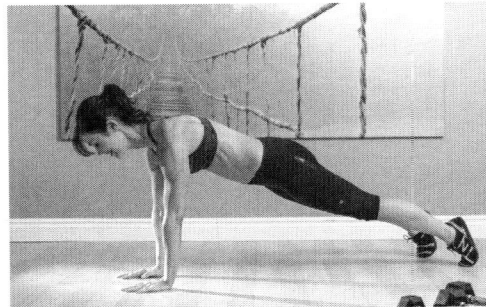

FRONT SQUATS

Appears in: Killer #4; Super Pump #2
Targeted Muscles: Front & back of legs; Buttocks; Shoulders; Abdominals

Stand with your feet shoulder-width apart. Holding a dumbbell in each hand, lift each weight up so that they are parallel to the floor and the ends are in line with the front of your shoulders. With your head and chest up, slowly bend at the hips and knees into a squat position. Keep your knees overtop of your ankles so that your knees do not pass too far over your toes. Stand up by pushing through the heels of your feet.

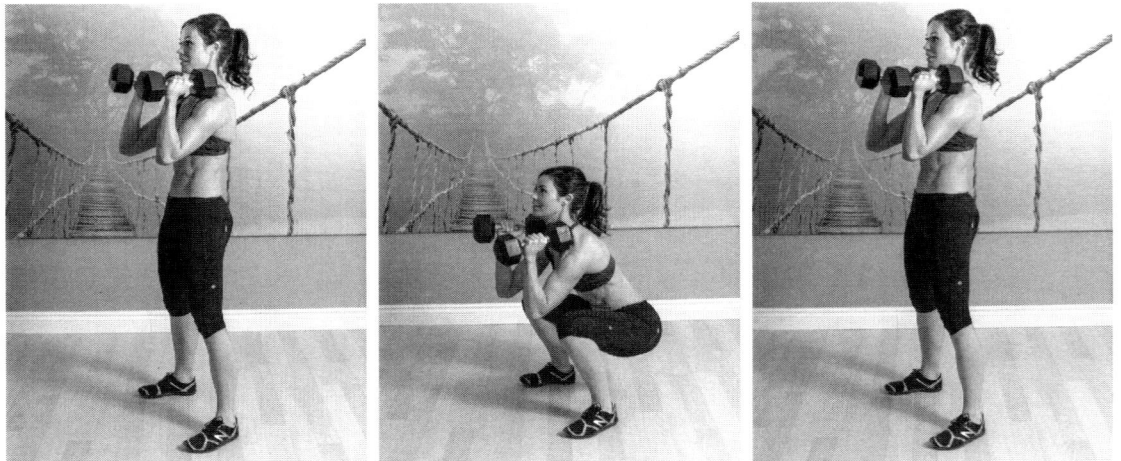

HIGH KNEES

Appears in: Super Pump #2; Sweaty Intervals #1, #2, #3, #4
Targeted Muscles: Front & back of legs; Abdominals; Calves; Your heart!

Hold your hands out in front of you at waist height. Quickly jump, one leg up at a time, high enough to hit your hand with your knee. Keep your chest up high during the entire movement. Repeat as quickly as you can for the specified amount of time.

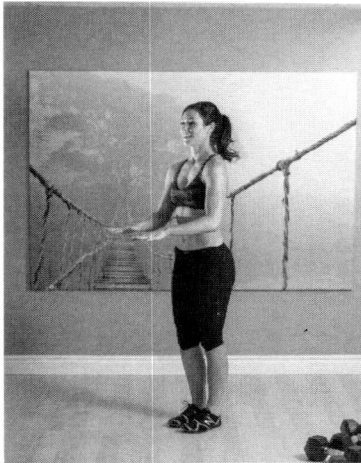

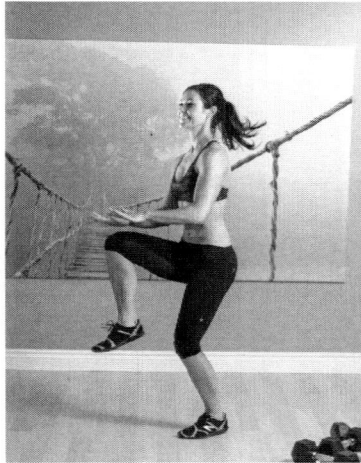

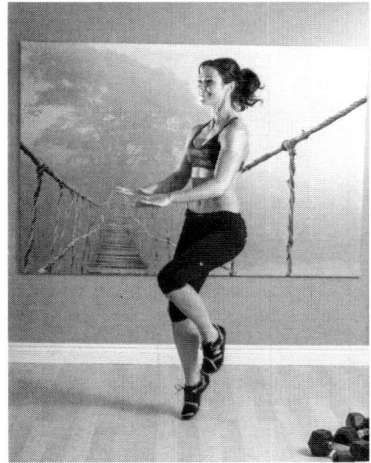

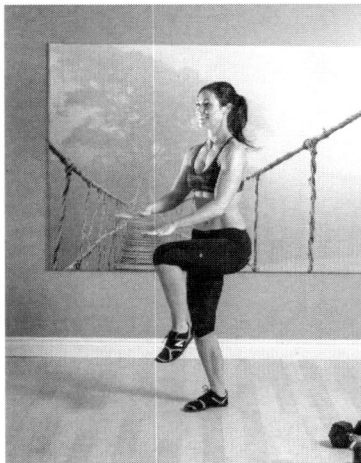

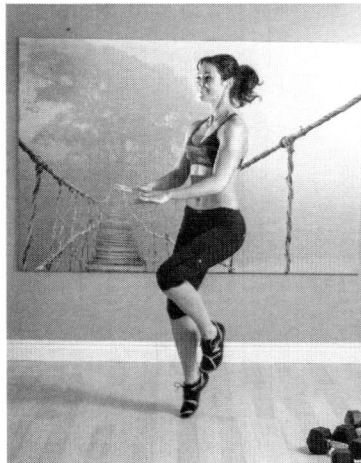

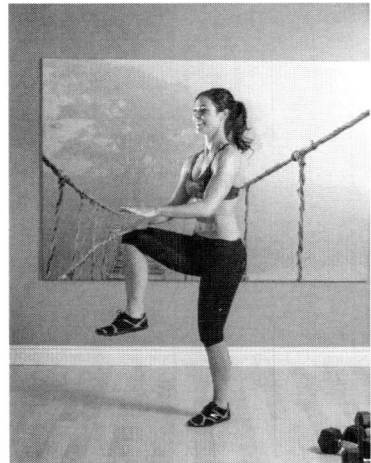

JACKS

Appears in: Super Pump #1; Sweaty Intervals #1, #2, #3, #4
Targeted Muscles: Legs; Buttocks; Shoulders; Abdominals; Your heart!

Jump your feet outside of shoulder-width apart as you raise your arms up and out at the same time by your sides. Jump your feet back into centre and bring your arms around and down simultaneously. Repeat this movement as quickly as you can for the specified amount of time.

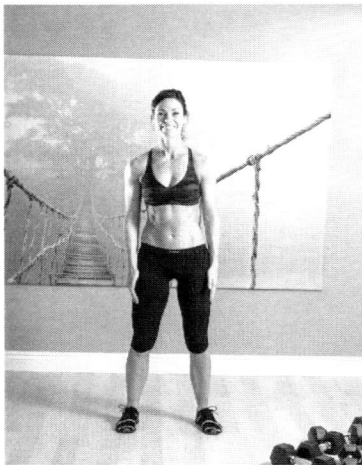

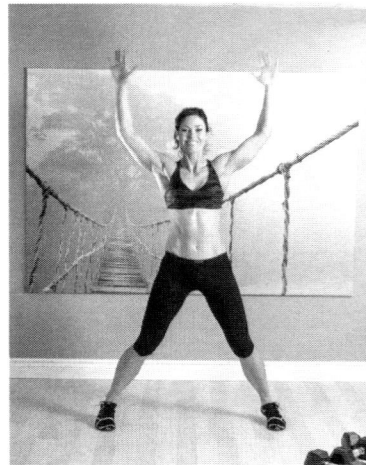

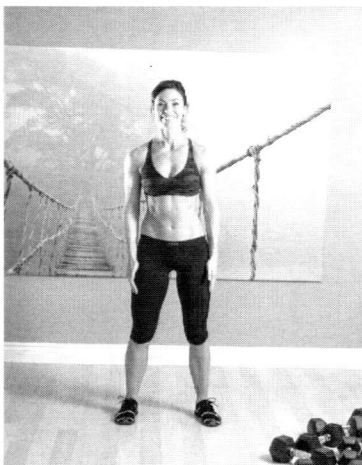

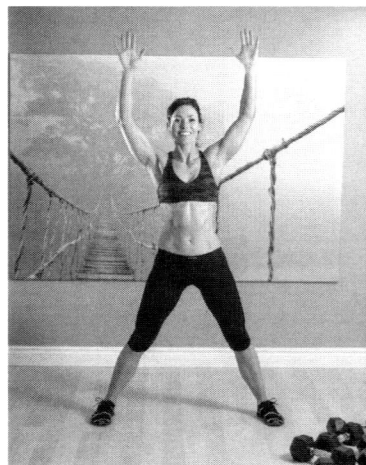

JUMP SQUATS

Appears in: Killer #6; Super Pump #3
Targeted Muscles: Front & back of legs; Buttocks; Abdominals; Your heart!

Start with your feet shoulder-width apart. Bend down into a squat (keeping your knees over your ankles and your chest up) and leap from this position up off the floor, catching yourself as you come down into another squat.

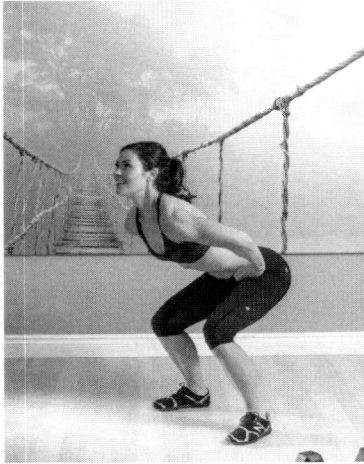

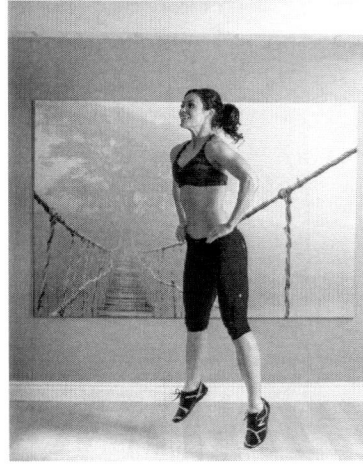

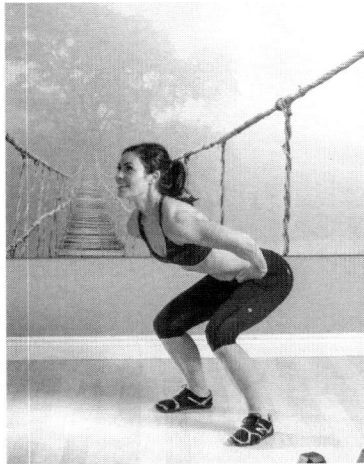

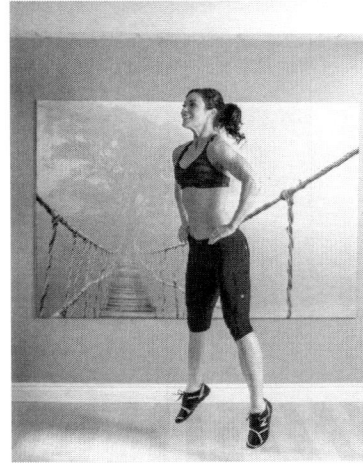

JUMPING JACK PLANKS

Appears in: Sweaty Intervals #3, #4
Targeted Muscles: Shoulders; Abdominals; Upper back; Your heart!

From a plank position (see Base Plank to review), quickly jump both of your feet simultaneously outward to shoulder-width apart then back to centre. Continue this jumping movement as quickly as you can for the specified amount of time.

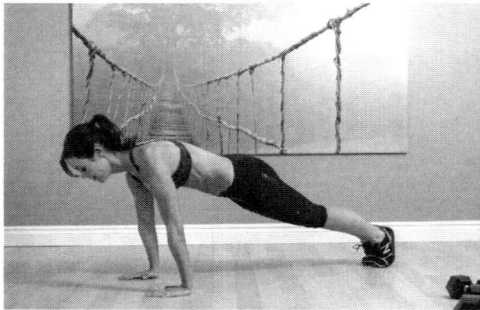

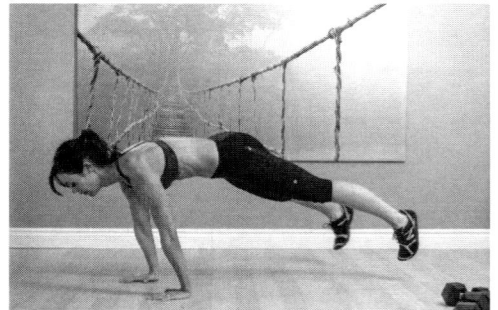

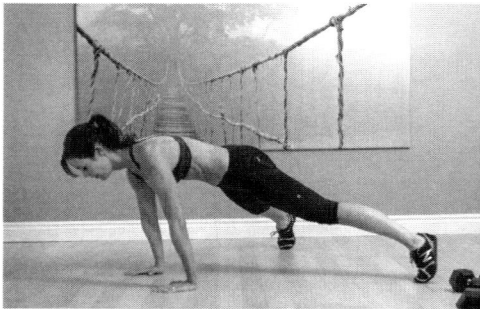

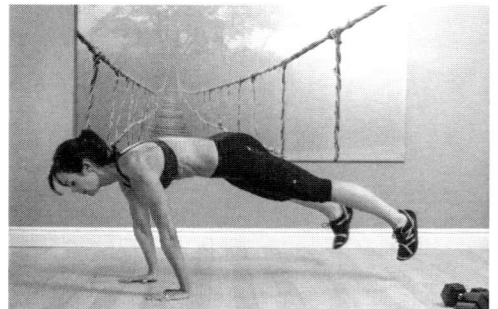

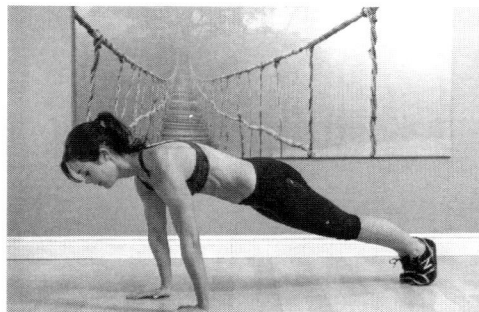

JUMPS WITH FOOT TOUCHES IN THE AIR

Appears in: Super Pump #4
Targeted Muscles: Calves; Legs; Abdominals; Your heart!

Start with your feet shoulder-width apart. Jump into the air and quickly touch or kick your feet together before you land on the ground again with feet still shoulder-width apart. Repeat as quickly as you can for the specified amount of time.

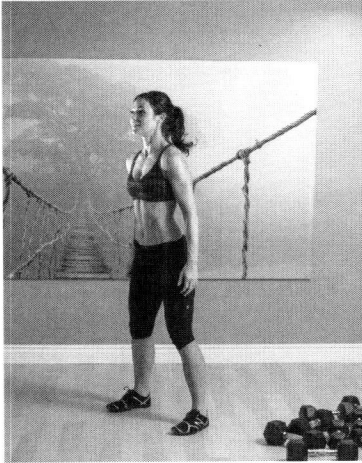

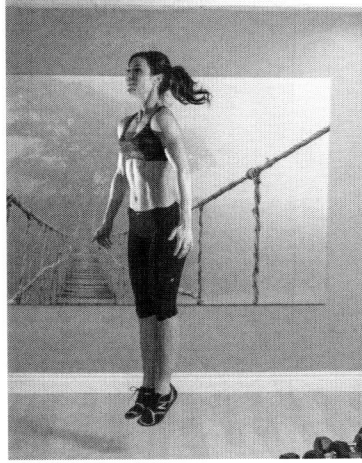

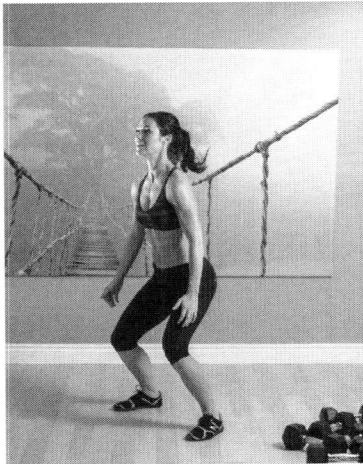

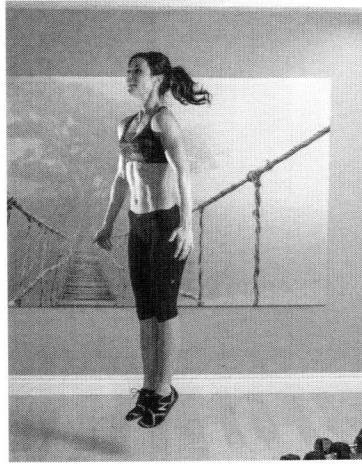

KNEE TO ELBOW PUSHUPS (PHOTOS ON NEXT PAGE)

Appears in: Killer #6
Targeted Muscles: Shoulders; Abdominals; Chest; Side of torso

In a plank position, place your hands just slightly wider than shoulder-width apart. With a tight core, crunch your right knee up to the outside of your right elbow, then step the leg back and repeat the crunch with your left knee to your left elbow. From here, complete one pushup by slowly lowering your body weight down in a straight line so your shoulders and hips move at the same rate. Your chest should fall between your hands. Go as low as you can without resting on the floor, pause, then push yourself back up to the starting position. Complete the series (one crunch to right elbow, back, one crunch to left elbow, back, pushup) for the specified number of repetitions.

KNEE TO ELBOW PUSHUPS (CONTINUED)

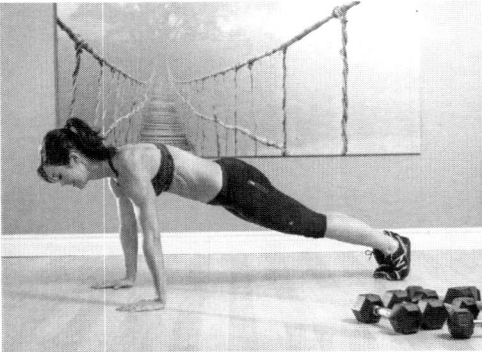

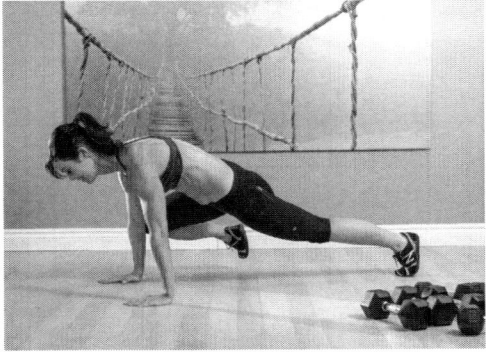

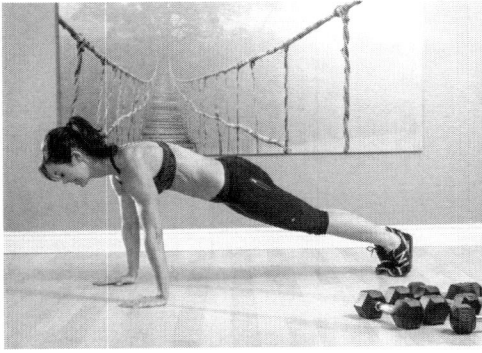

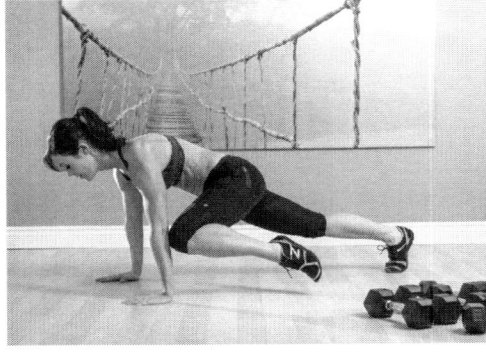

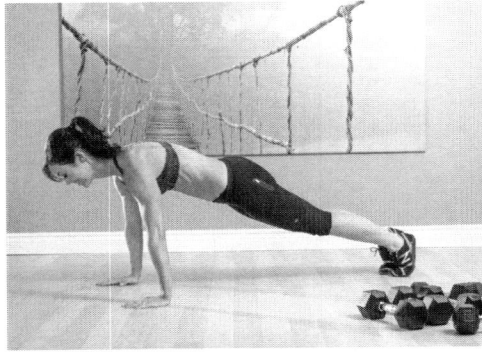

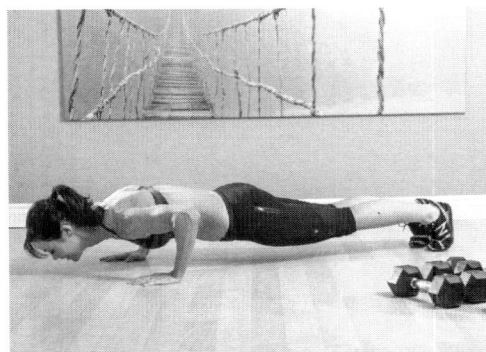

LATERAL RAISES WITH ¼ LUNGE

Appears in: Killer #1
Targeted Muscles: Side of shoulders; Front of legs; Abdominals; Upper back

With one weight in each hand, take a large step forward and bend both of your knees so that you are ¼ of the way down to the floor. With tall posture, slowly raise both of your arms up to your sides, no higher than shoulder height. (Keep your shoulder blades down your back. You will know you are in the correct position if you start the exercise by lifting your shoulders up, back, and down. This is called the shoulder set position). Pause with the dumbbells at your side for a brief moment before slowly lowering the weights back down.

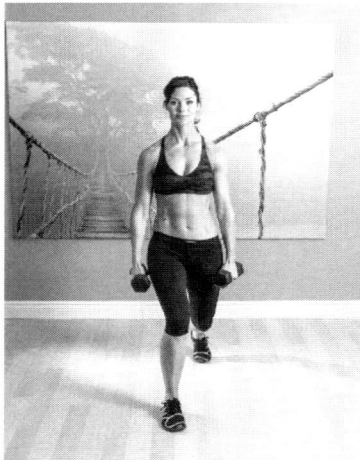

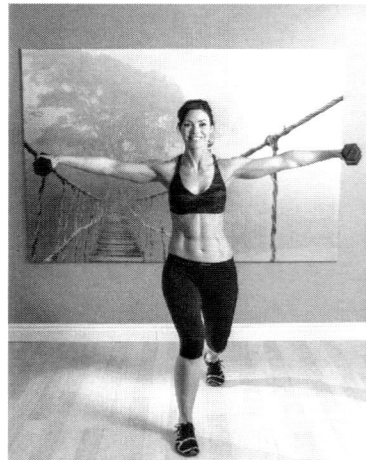

LATERAL SHUFFLE

Appears in: Killer #2; Super Pump #1
Targeted Muscles: Sides of legs; Buttocks; Calves; Your heart!

You will need space such as a hallway to perform this exercise, as you will be covering a little distance with each step to the side. From a standing position, take a lateral (sideways) step to the right with your right foot. Carry your left foot in to replace where your right foot was. While pushing off with the left foot, take another lateral step with your right foot. Continue this pattern until the edge of your space and then repeat in the opposite direction. Think of this exercise as running sideways! Complete for the specified amount of time.

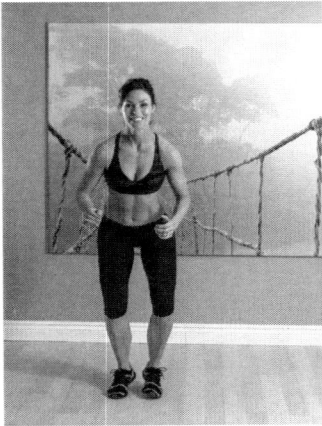

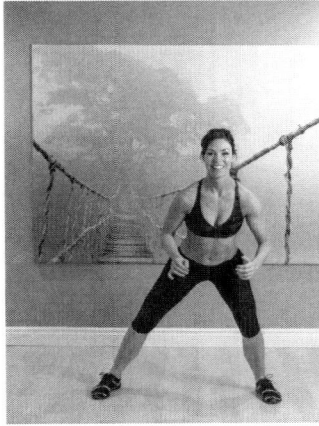

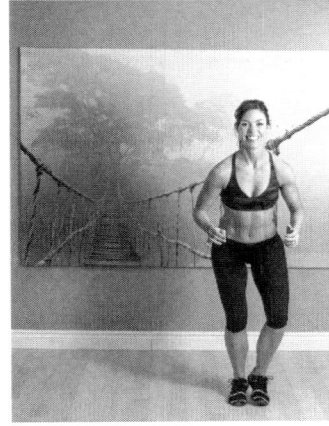

LAWNMOWER

Appears in: Killer #4, #8
Targeted Muscles: Front, back, & inner legs; Front & back of arms; Front & back of shoulders; Buttocks; Mid-back; Side of torso

From standing and with a weight in front of you, take a large step to one side so that your feet are wider than shoulder-width apart. Keep both of your feet facing forward. Leaning to one side, slowly bend at one hip, pushing your body weight back onto your heel while you bend your one knee. Keep your other leg straight (side lunge position). Rest your elbow on your bent knee and pull a weight with the other hand upward in the direction of the armpit to mimic the motion of pulling a lawnmower cord. Be sure your head turns in the same direction as your arm to protect your neck from kinking. Complete the specified repetitions on one side, then switch to the other side.

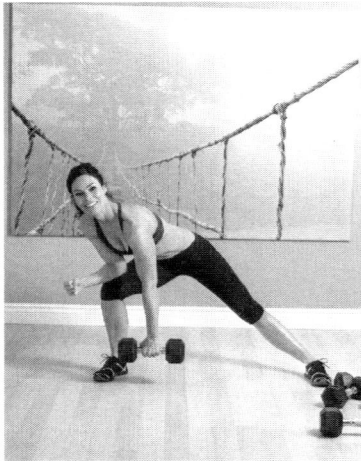

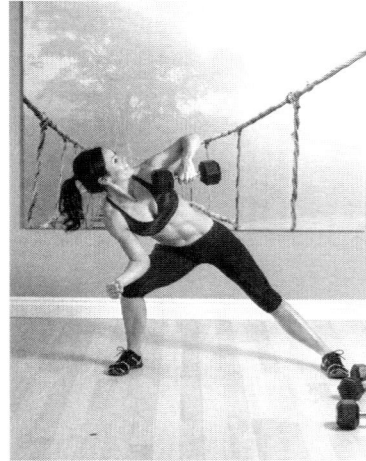

MID ROW (PALMS FACING UPWARD)

Appears in: Killer #6; Super Pump #3
Targeted Muscles: Front & back of arms; Shoulders; Upper back; Abdominals

With a weight in each hand, palms facing away from you, stand with your feet shoulder-width apart. Bend your knees and flex your torso forward (keep your back flat). Squeeze your buttocks to maintain a strong core, and keep your weight in your heels. Slowly bring both weights up toward your rib cage and away from your thighs, then slowly lower back down.

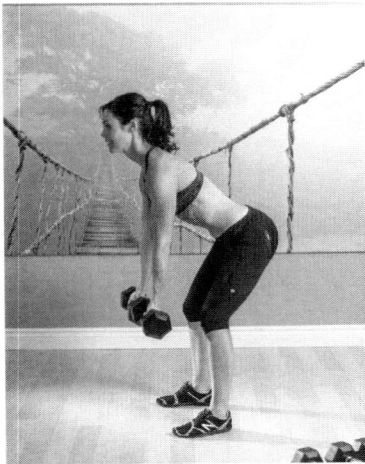

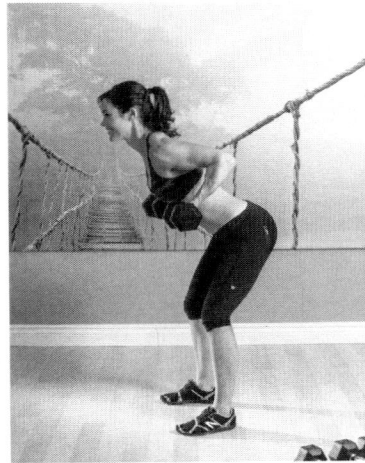

OBLIQUE CRUNCH OFF BALL

Appears in: Killer #5
Targeted Muscles: Side of torso

Place your hip on the side of an exercise ball and your feet against a solid surface with your bottom foot forward. Put your hands behind your head to open up your chest, and slowly bend upward pushing your hip into the ball and reaching your elbow sideways, tracking over the side of your torso. Your shoulder, hip, and feet should remain in a straight line even when you are crunching upwards. Complete the specified repetitions on one side, then repeat on the other side.

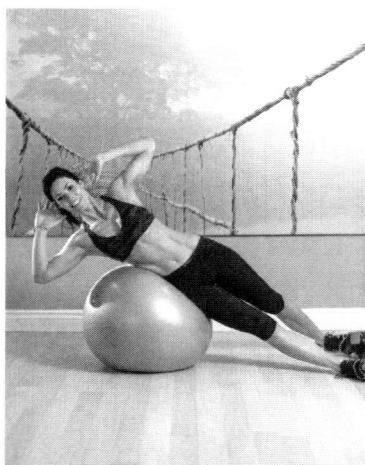

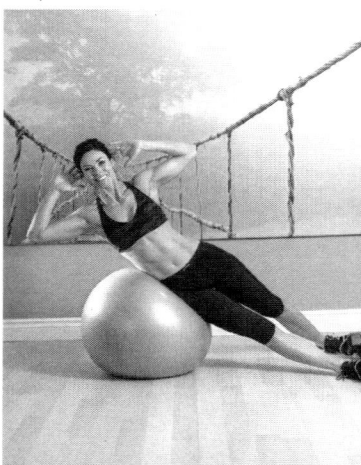

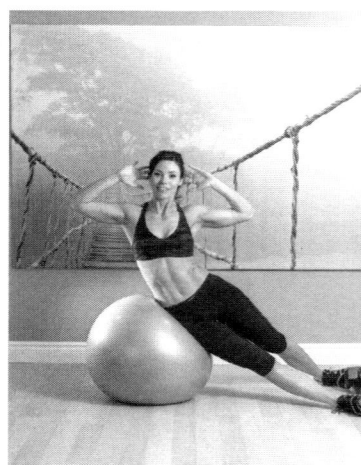

PIKE/PLANK

Appears in: Killer #4
Targeted Muscles: Shoulders; Abdominals; Mid-back; Upper back

Start in a plank position on your toes and with both hands directly under your shoulders. Keep your hips flat for a two second count. From there, push back with the heels of your hands and slowly raise your hips up into the air as high as you can, while maintaining balance on your toes. Pause in this top position for two seconds then go back into the starting plank position.

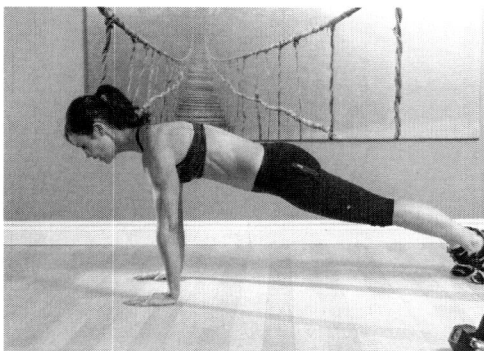

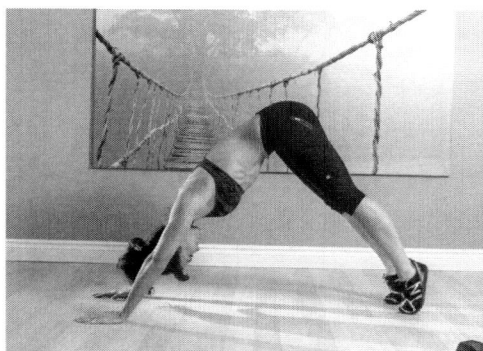

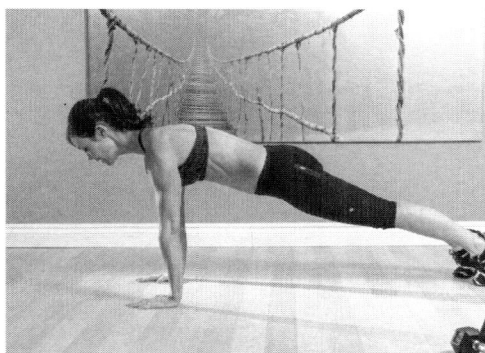

PLANK OFF BALL

Appears in: Killer #5; Super Pump #3
Targeted Muscles: Upper back; Shoulders; Abdominals

Place both of your elbows directly underneath your shoulders onto an exercise ball. Extend one leg out at a time to form a plank position. With a tight core (tilt your tailbone toward the floor), hold this position for the specified amount of time.

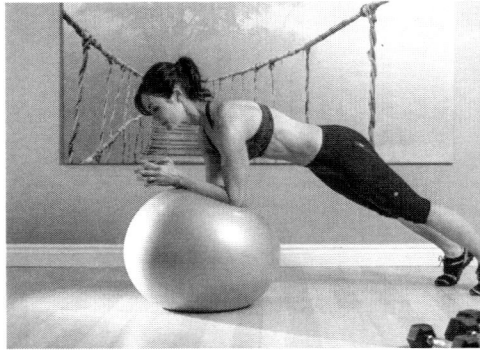

PLANK OFF BALL WITH PRESS-OUTS

Appears in: Killer #7; Super Pump #4
Targeted Muscles: Upper back; Shoulders; Abdominals

Place both of your elbows directly underneath your shoulders onto an exercise ball. Extend one leg out at a time to form a plank position. With a tight core (tilt your tailbone toward the floor), slowly push the ball forward and back 2-3 inches underneath your body weight. Keep your body as still as possible as you move your arms.

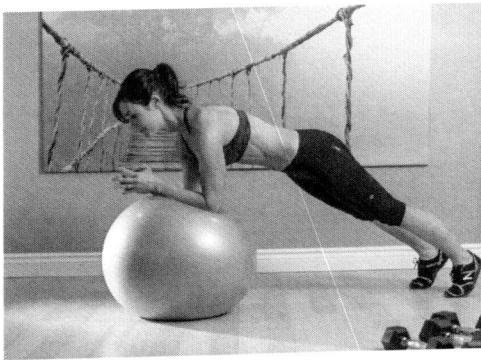

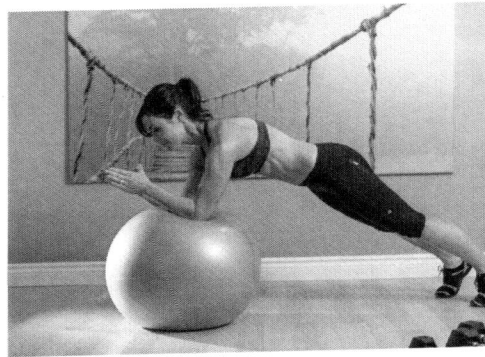

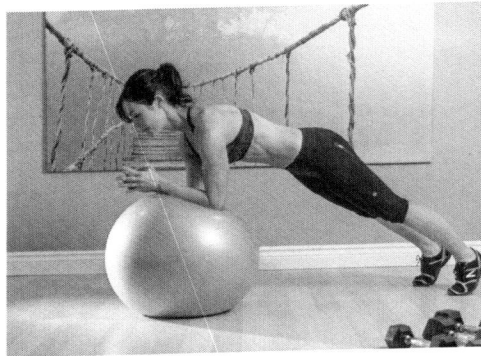

PLANK OFF FOREARMS

Appears in: Killer #1; Super Pump #1
Targeted Muscles: Upper back; Shoulders; Abdominals

Lying on your stomach, place your forearms on the floor with your elbows directly under your shoulders. Lift your body up off the floor using the pressure from your arms and your toes. Tilt your tailbone toward the floor (as if you were slightly tucking your buttocks underneath you). This helps to isolate your abdominal muscles. Hold this position for the specified amount of time.

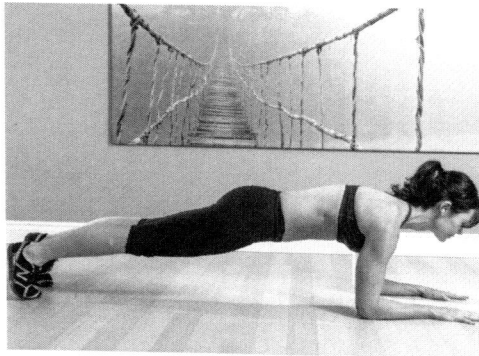

PLANK WITH ALTERNATING ROW

Appears in: Killer #6; Super Pump #3
Targeted Muscles: Front & back of arms; Shoulders; Abdominals; Upper back

Start in a plank position on your toes, with your hands directly underneath your shoulders, and with a weight/dumbbell on the floor beneath your chest. Keeping a tight core (tilt your tailbone toward the floor), slowly grasp the weight underneath your chest and row it up (pull) toward your rib cage while keeping your hips as still as possible (the less rocking from side to side, the more you will get out of this exercise). Slowly lower the weight to the floor, then let go and grab the weight with the other hand and row up to the other side of your body.

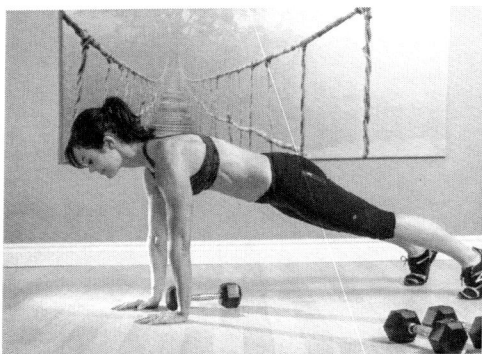

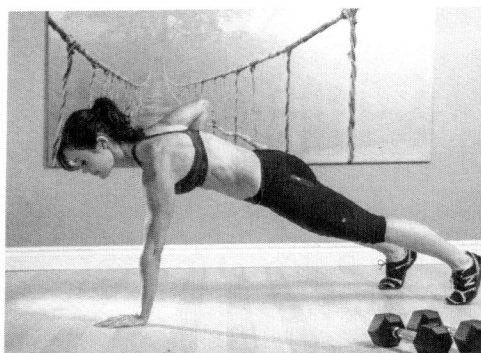

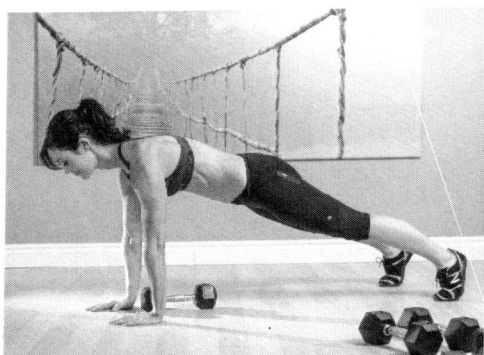

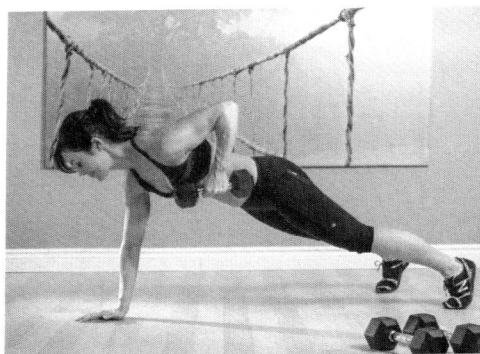

PLANK WITH WEIGHT SLIDE (PHOTOS ON NEXT PAGE)

Appears in: Killer #8
Targeted Muscles: Shoulders; Abdominals; Upper back

Place a weight plate or dumbbell in a towel so that it will slide easily across the floor.

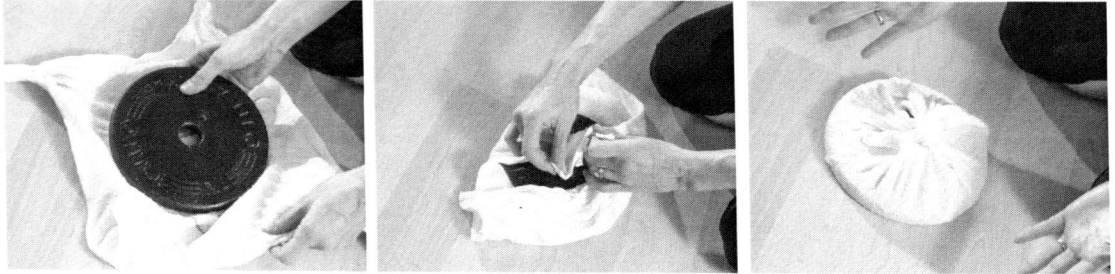

From a plank position off your elbows (see "Base Plank" to review), reach out and grasp the weight in the towel. Slowly slide it around your balancing elbow. Leave the weight at that elbow and then switch arms so that you can grab the weight and slide it around the opposite elbow. Keep your hips as still as possible to get the most out of this exercise.

PLANK WITH WEIGHT SLIDE (CONTINUED)

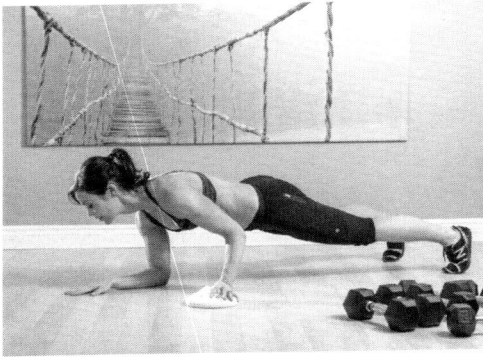

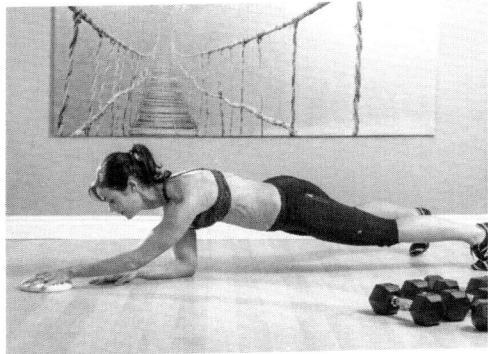

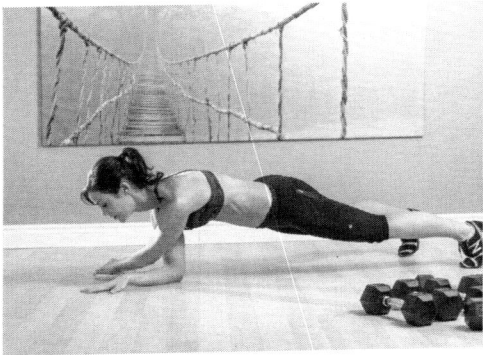

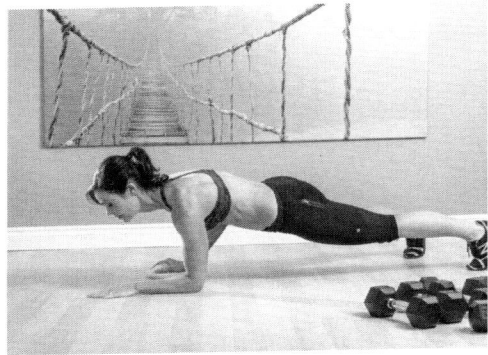

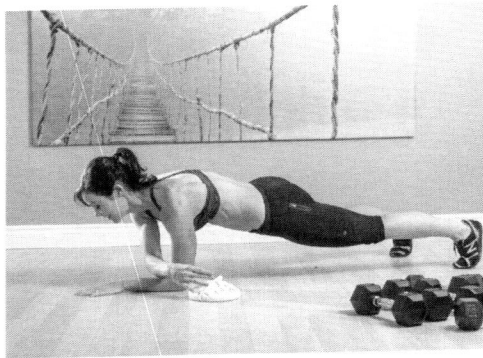

PUSHUPS OFF ELEVATED SURFACE

Appears in: Killer #7
Targeted Muscles: Abdominals; Upper back; Chest; Shoulders

Place your toes on an elevated, stable surface (bench, chair, stair). Place your hands just slightly wider than shoulder-width apart. With a tight core (as if you were slightly tucking your buttocks underneath you), slowly lower your body weight down in a straight line so your shoulders and hips move at the same rate. Your chest should fall between your hands. Go as low as you can without resting on the floor, pause, then push yourself back up to the starting position.

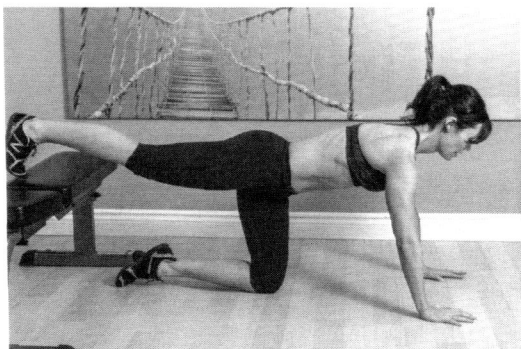

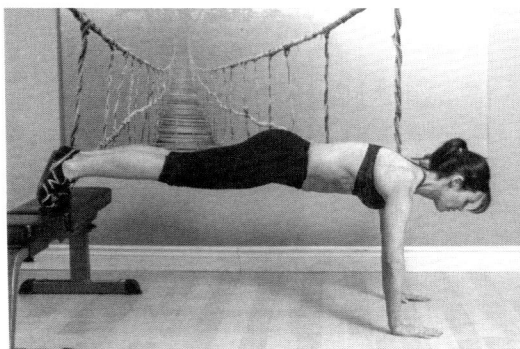

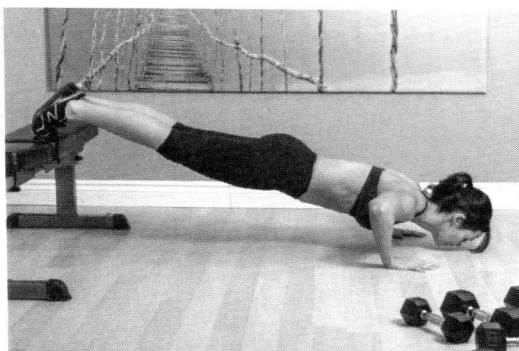

PUSHUPS OFF KNEES

Appears in: Killer #1; Super Pump #1
Targeted Muscles: Abdominals; Upper back; Chest; Shoulders

Lie face down on the floor with your hands shoulder-width or just outside shoulder-width apart. Bend your knees, keeping your feet on the floor, as you raise your body up off the floor until your arms are straight. Keep your body straight and slowly bend your elbows at a 45-degree angle to lower your body weight back down to the floor, leading with your chest. Your hips and chest should move at the same rate, and your body position should be rigid as you pivot on your knees toward the floor. Pause at the bottom, and then push through your hands until your arms are straight again.

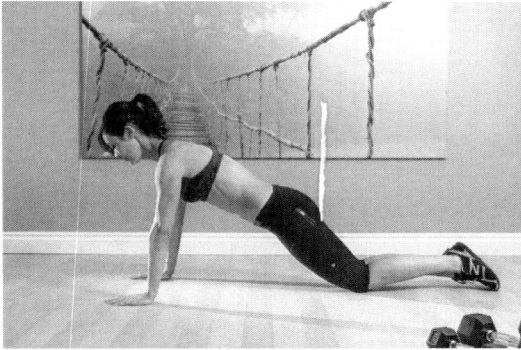

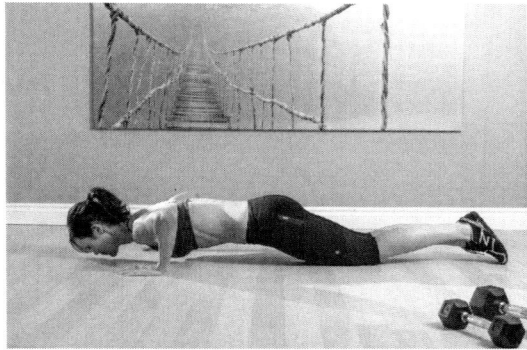

PUSHUPS OFF TOES

Appears in: Killer #4
Targeted Muscles: Abdominals; Upper back; Chest; Shoulders

Lie face down on the floor with your hands shoulder-width or just outside shoulder-width apart. Curl your toes under and lift your body up into a plank position off your hands. Keep your body straight and slowly bend your elbows at a 45-degree angle to lower your body weight back down to the floor, leading with your chest. Your hips and chest should move at the same rate, and your body position should be rigid as you pivot off your toes toward the floor. Pause at the bottom, and then push through your hands until your arms are straight again.

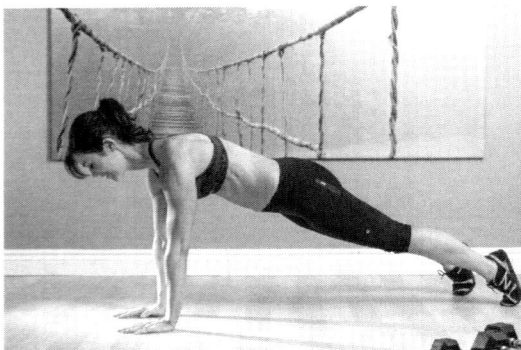

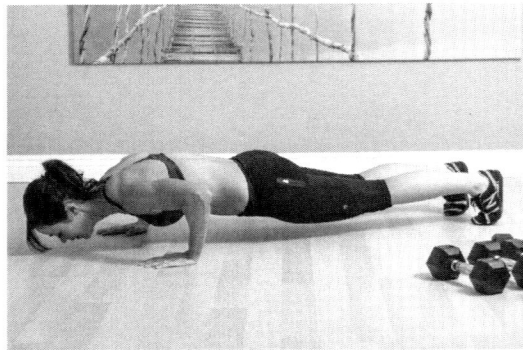

PUSHUPS OFF TOES, ONE LEG ELEVATED

Appears in: Super Pump #4
Targeted Muscles: Abdominals; Upper back; Chest; Shoulders; Buttocks

Start in a plank position off your toes with your hands just slightly wider than shoulder-width apart. With a tight core, raise one leg up while keeping the buttock contracted, and then slowly lower your body weight down in a straight line so your shoulders and hips move at the same rate. Your chest should fall between your hands. Go as low as you can without resting on the floor, pause, then push yourself back up to the starting position. Alternate each leg lift between pushups.

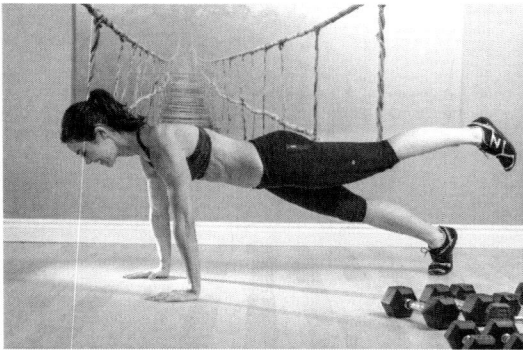

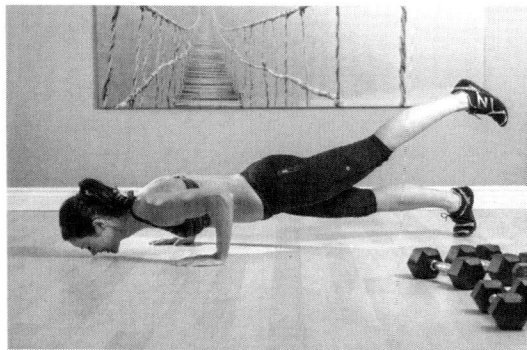

REAR DELT FLYS

Appears in: Killer #3
Targeted Muscles: Upper back; Back of shoulders

Hold two dumbbells below your chest (hands facing thighs). Bend at the hips and slightly in the knees, maintaining a straight/flat back. Slowly raise your arms up to your sides (shoulder height) with your elbows slightly bent. It is important you see the weights in your peripheral vision so you know you are not raising the weights too far behind you. Pause at shoulder height for one second, and then lower both arms back down below your chest.

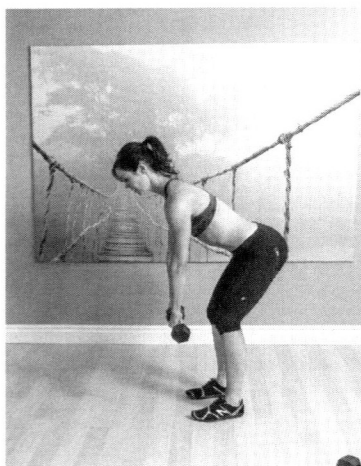

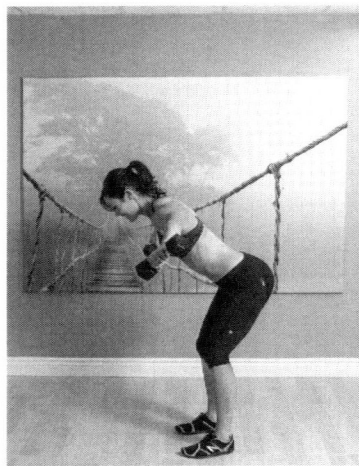

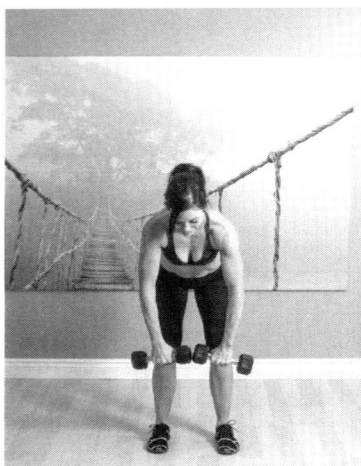

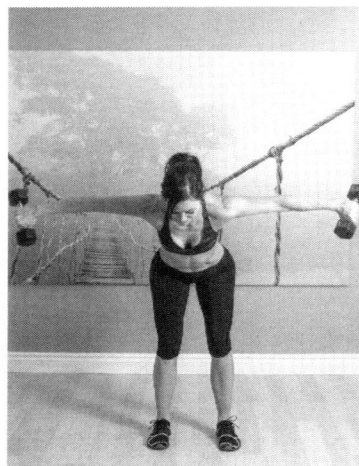

SHOULDER PRESS

Appears in: Killer #1
Targeted Muscles: Shoulders; Abdominals

Stand with your feet shoulder-width apart and your knees slightly bent. Lift your dumbbells to shoulder height so both your arms start at your sides forming a 90-degree angle at your elbows. Slowly and simultaneously push the dumbbells upward over your head so that they touch in the centre, then lower your arms back down to 90 degrees.

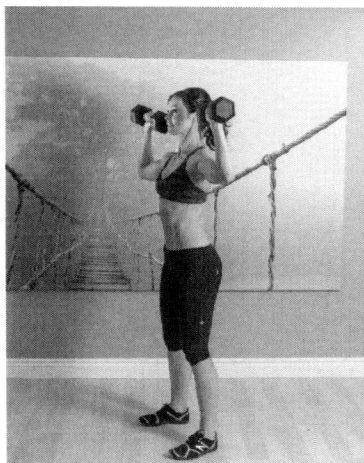

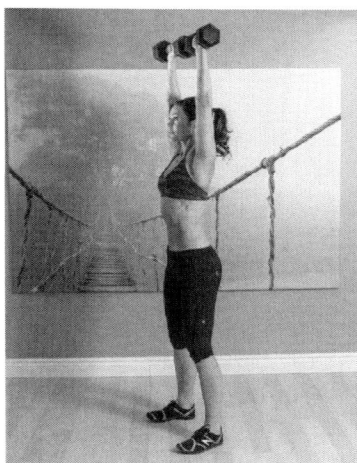

SIDE LUNGES (DYNAMIC)

Appears in: Killer #5
Targeted Muscles: Front, back, & inner legs; Calves; Buttocks; Abdominals;
Upper back; Shoulders

Take a large step to one side so that your feet are wider than shoulder-width apart. Keep both of your feet facing forward. On one side, slowly bend at the hip and push your body weight back onto your heel while you bend your knee, keeping your other leg straight. Push yourself back up into a standing position (using the bent leg) so that your feet meet back in the middle. Complete the specified number of repetitions on one side, then switch to the other side.

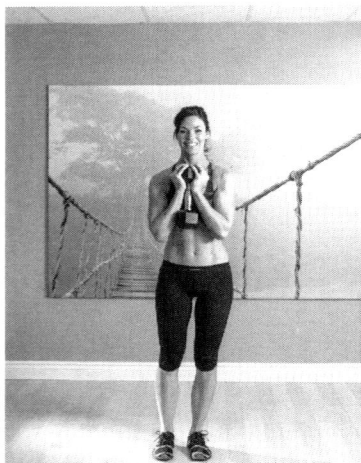

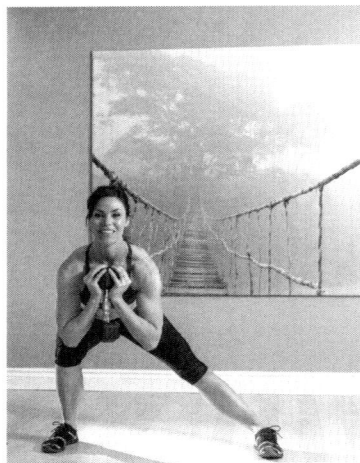

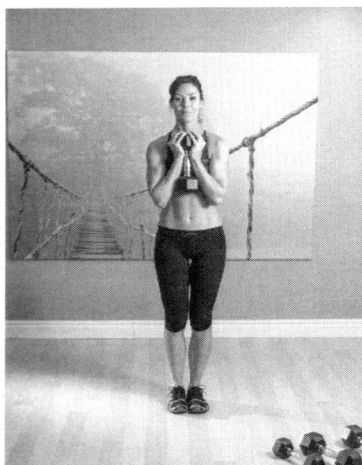

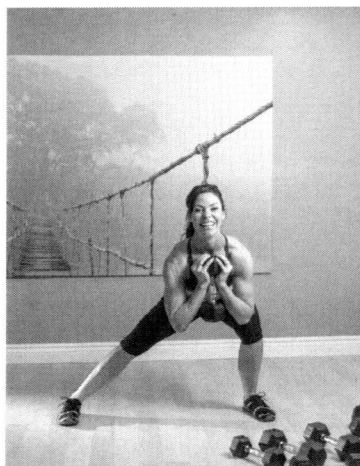

SIDE LUNGES (STATIC)

Appears in: Killer #3; Super Pump #2
Targeted Muscles: Front, back, & inner legs; Buttocks

Take a large step to one side so that your feet are wider than shoulder-width apart. Keep both of your feet facing forward. On one side, slowly bend at the hip and push your body weight back onto your heel while you bend your knee, keeping your other leg straight. Push yourself back up into a standing position (using the bent leg). Note that your feet do not move during this exercise (which is why it is called "Static"). Complete the specified repetitions on one side, then switch to the other side.

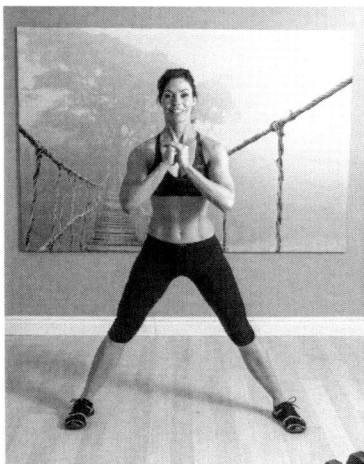

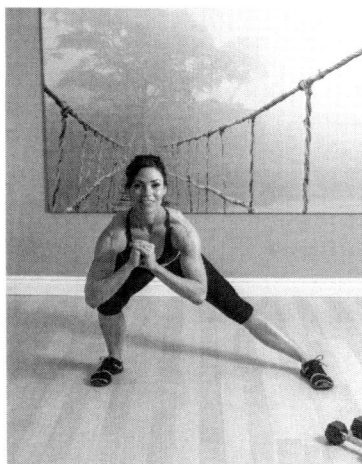

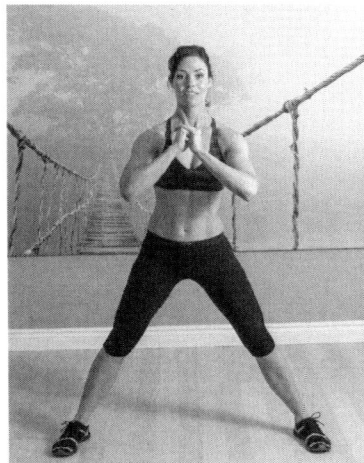

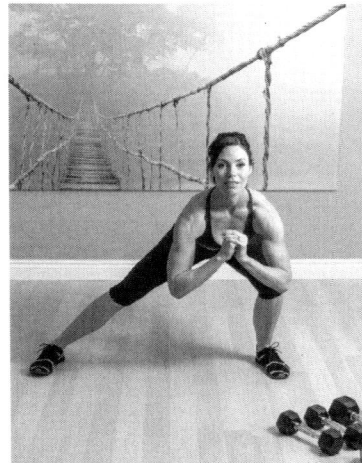

SIDE PLANK OFF TOES

Appears in: Killer #3; Super Pump #2
Targeted Muscles: Side of torso; Upper back; Shoulders

Lie on your side and extend your legs outward. Your feet, hips, and shoulders should be in a straight line. Place your bottom elbow directly underneath your shoulder, and keep your bottom hand on the floor facing perpendicular to your body. Using your oblique muscles (the sides of your torso) and a little pressure from your balancing elbow and the side of your foot, slowly raise your body weight up, keeping your hips off the floor. From here, raise your top arm straight up so that your shoulders are in line. Hold this position for the specified amount of time, and then switch sides.

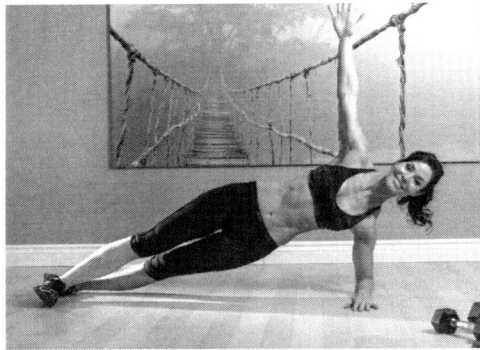

SIDE PLANK OFF KNEES

Appears in: Killer #2
Targeted Muscles: Shoulders; Side of torso; Upper back

Lying on your side, bend your legs at the knees behind you at a 90-degree angle. Keep your knees, hips, and shoulders in a straight line. Place your bottom elbow directly underneath your shoulder, and keep your bottom hand on the floor, perpendicular to your body. Using your oblique muscles (the sides of your torso) and a little pressure through your bottom elbow and bottom knee, lift your hips and upper body off the floor. From there, raise your top arm straight up so that your shoulders are in line. Hold this position for the specified amount of time, and then repeat on the other side of your body.

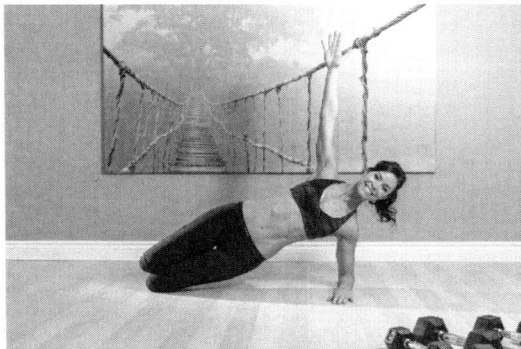

SIDE PLANK WITH ARM ROTATIONS
(PHOTOS ON NEXT PAGE)

Appears in: Killer #6, #8
Targeted Muscles: Side of torso; Shoulders; Abdominals; Upper back

Lie on your side and extend your legs outward. Your feet, hips, and shoulders should be in a straight line. Place your bottom elbow directly underneath your shoulder, keeping your bottom hand on the floor facing perpendicular to your body. Using your oblique muscles (the sides of your torso) and a little pressure from your balancing elbow and the outside of your foot, slowly raise your body weight up and lift your hips off the floor. Raise your top arm up and clasp your hand behind your head. From here, gently lead with your top (bent) elbow and rotate it toward the floor. Go as low as your body will allow, pause, then rotate back up to the starting position. Note that you are not reaching the elbow, you are just using it to gauge how far you rotate. All of the rotation should come from your torso, not your arm. Keep your elbow in line with your shoulder throughout the entire movement. Complete the specified repetitions on one side, then switch to the other side.

SIDE PLANK WITH ARM ROTATIONS
(CONTINUED)

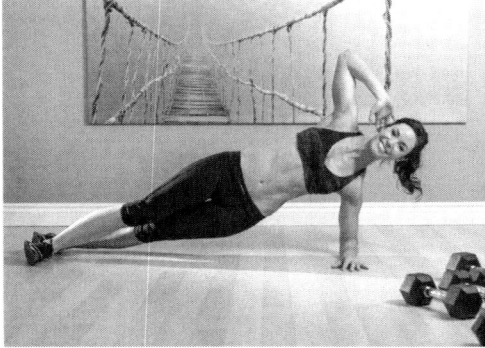

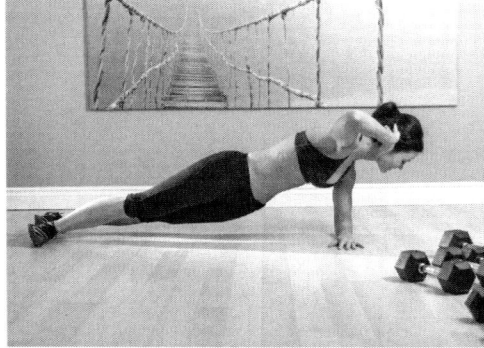

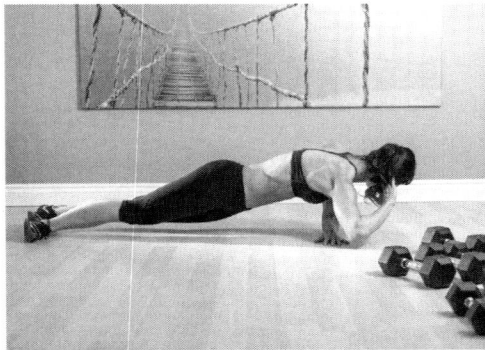

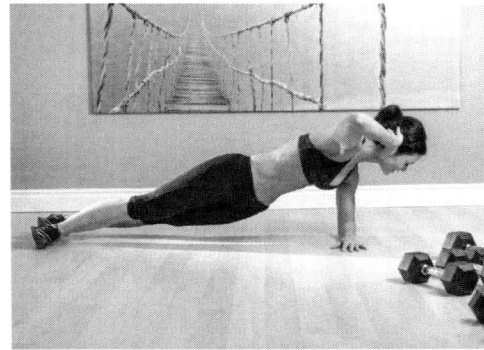

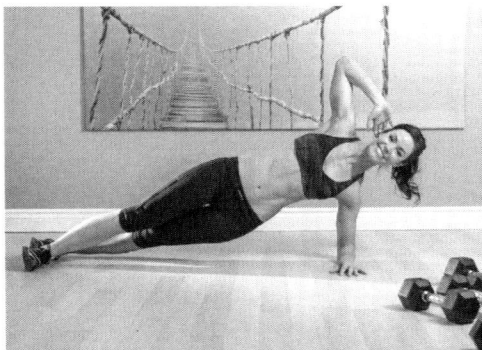

SIDE PLANK WITH TOP LEG LIFT

Appears in: Killer #7
Targeted Muscles: Side of torso; Buttocks; Shoulders; Abdominals; Upper back

Lie on your side and extend your legs outward. Your feet, hips, and shoulders should be in a straight line. Place your bottom elbow directly underneath your shoulder. Keep your bottom hand on the floor, perpendicular to your body. Using your oblique muscles (the sides of your torso) and a little pressure from your balancing elbow and the side of your foot, slowly raise your body weight up and lift your hips off the floor. Extend your top arm to form a T position with your body. From here slowly raise your top leg up as high as your body will allow, then lower without rotating or compromising the lift of your torso. Complete the specified repetitions on one side, then switch to the other side.

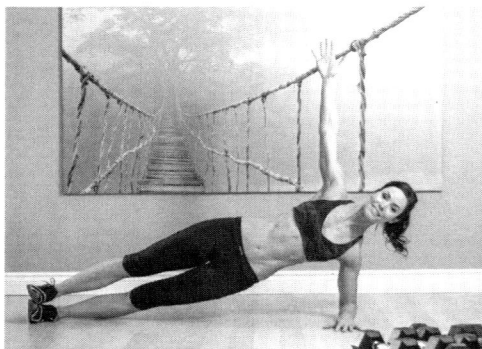

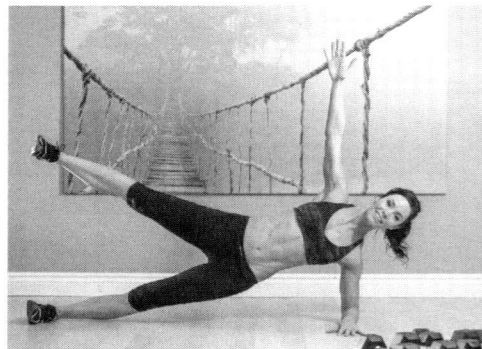

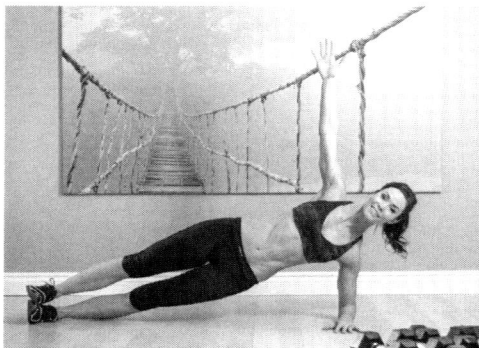

SIDE-TO-SIDE JUMP LUNGES

Appears in: Killer #7; Super Pump #4
Targeted Muscles: Front, back, & inner legs; Buttocks; Abdominals; Your heart!

From a standing position, take a large step to one side so that your feet are wider than shoulder-width apart. Keep both of your feet facing forward. Slowly bend at the hip and push your body weight back onto your heel while you bend your one knee. Keep your other leg straight. Push yourself back up to centre (a jumping motion) and continue into another side lunge on the opposite leg.

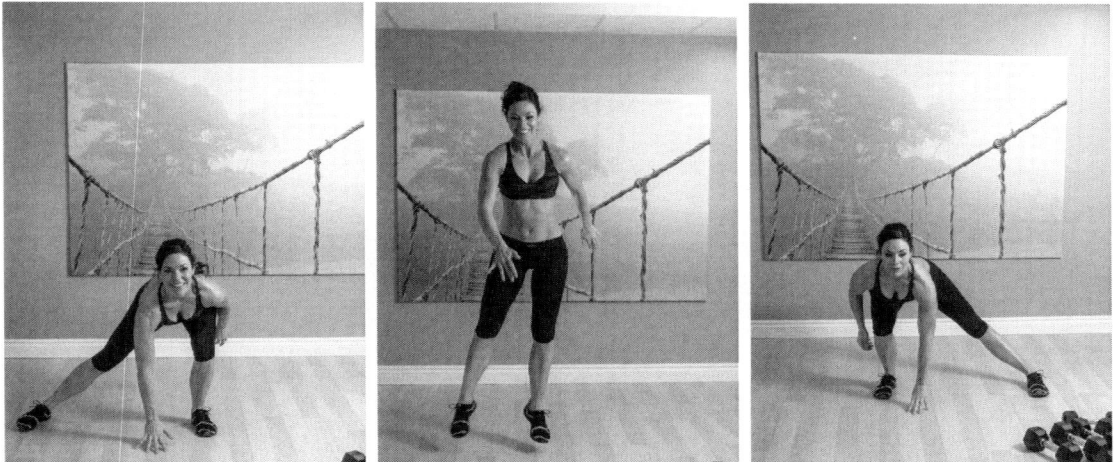

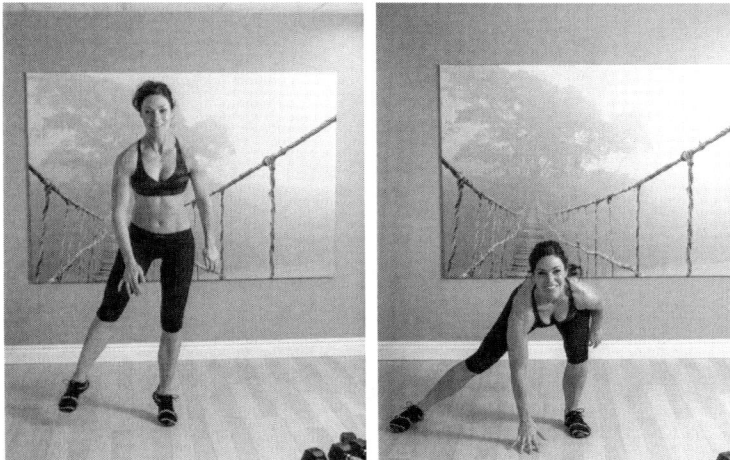

SINGLE ARM AND LEG SHOULDER PRESS

Appears in: Killer #8
Targeted Muscles: Shoulders; Abdominals; Buttocks; Calves

Stand with your feet shoulder-width apart and hold a weight in your right hand at your side. Lift your right leg up in front of you and then raise your right arm up to 90 degrees. Your standing leg and pressing arm are on opposite sides of your body. In this balanced position, slowly press the dumbbell up and down to 90 degrees for the specified number of repetitions. Repeat on the other side.

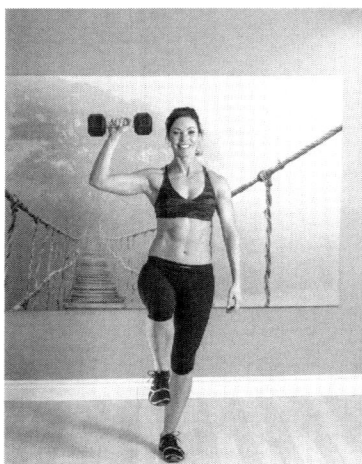

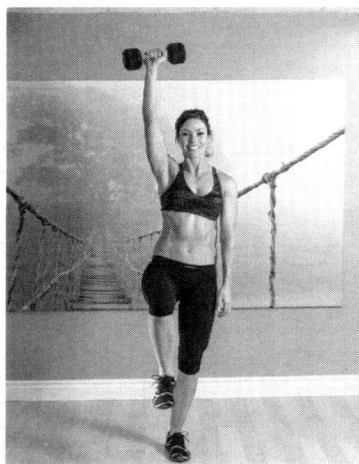

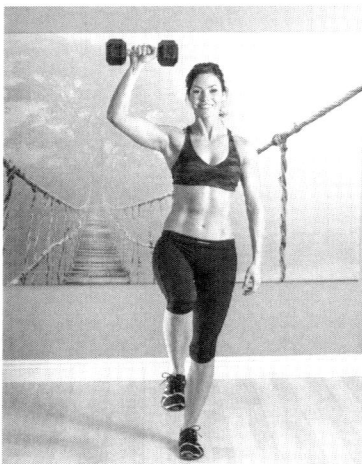

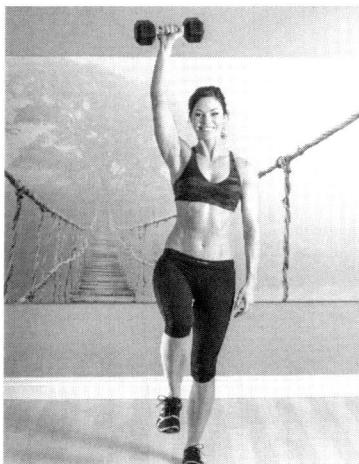

SINGLE LEG LATERAL RAISE

Appears in: Killer #6
Targeted Muscles: Side of shoulders; Abdominals; Buttocks; Calves; Upper back

Holding a weight in each hand, arms at your sides, balance on one foot and slowly raise both arms out to shoulder height (no higher) simultaneously. Keep your shoulder blades down your back as you raise your arms out to the side. This prevents you from raising your arms higher than shoulder height and engages your back muscles. Lower the weights back down to your hips. Complete the specified number of repetitions, then switch to balance on the other leg.

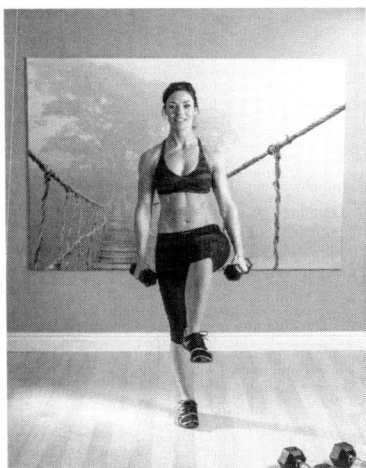

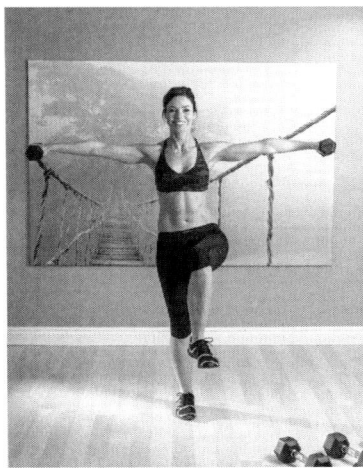

SINGLE LEG LUNGE WITH LATERAL TOUCH

Appears in: Killer #4
Targeted Muscles: Front & back of legs; Buttocks; Calves; Side of torso

Place the top of one foot on an elevated and stable surface (a bench, chair, stair). Take a large step forward with your other leg. Bend your front knee until your thigh is parallel to the floor (keep the pressure of your body weight in the heel of your balancing foot, not your toe). Slowly reach your hand around your knee and touch the lateral side (outside) of your balancing foot, then stand back up. Complete the specified number of repetitions, then switch to the other leg.

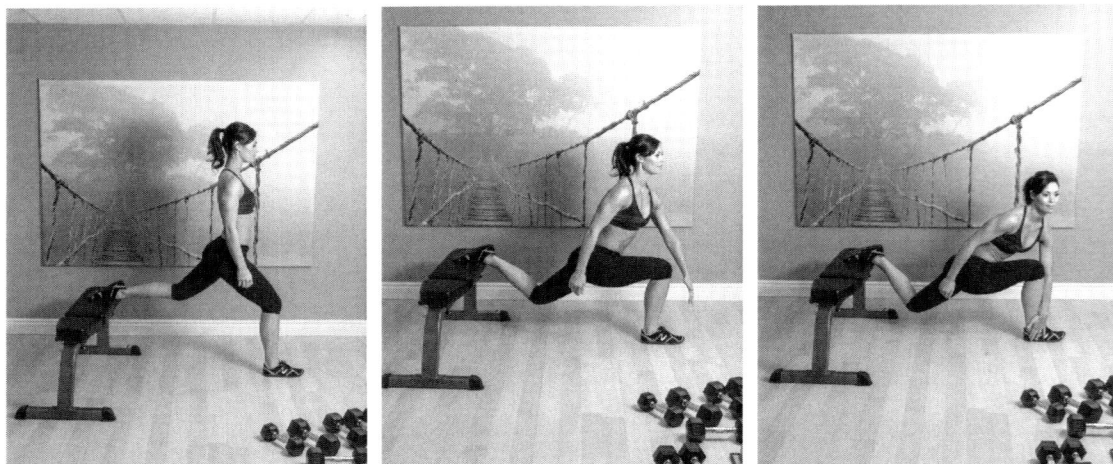

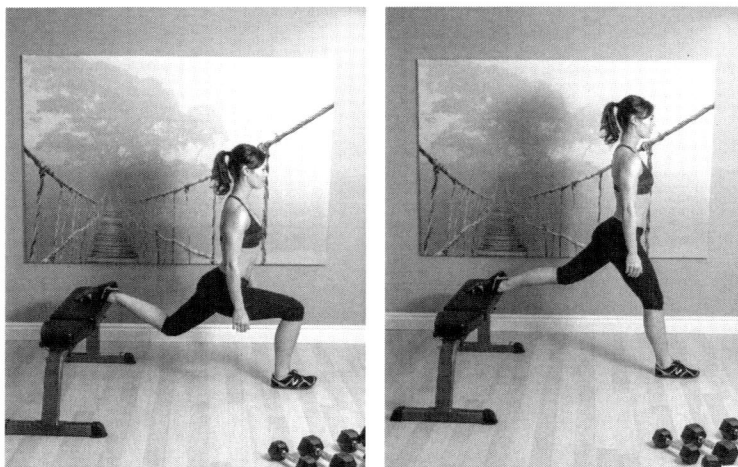

SINGLE LEG LUNGE WITH WEIGHT

Appears in: Killer #8
Targeted Muscles: Front & back of legs; Buttocks; Abdominals

Holding a dumbbell in each hand, reach back with one leg and place the top of your foot on an elevated and stable surface (a bench, chair, stair). Take a large step forward with your other leg. Bend your front knee until your thigh is parallel to the floor, and then stand back up by pushing through the heel of your balancing/front foot. Keep your knee tracking over your ankle rather than over your front toe. Complete the specified number of repetitions, then switch to the other leg.

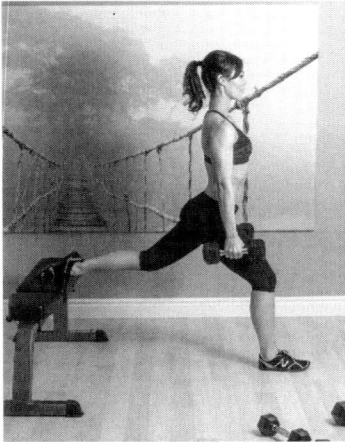

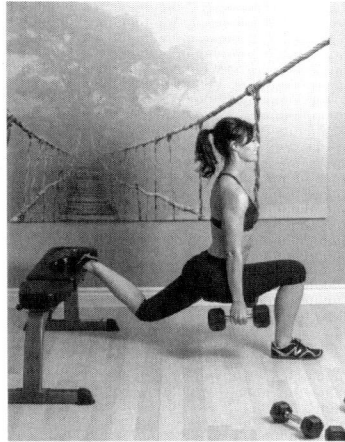

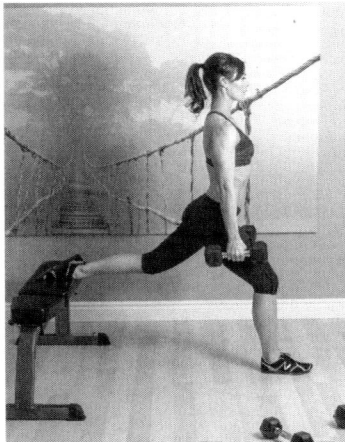

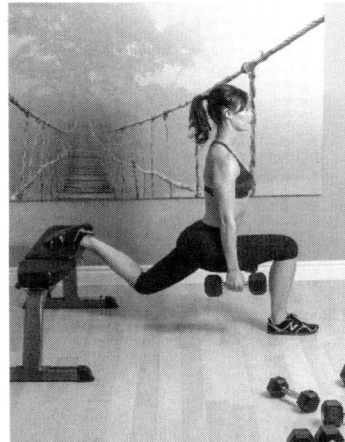

SINGLE LEG ROMANIAN DEADLIFTS

Appears in: Killer #3
Targeted Muscles: Upper back; Front & back of legs; Buttocks; Calves

Stand with your feet shoulder-width apart and with your hands in front of your thighs (wrists facing each other). Holding a weight in each hand, lift one leg back and upward as you simultaneously drop your torso forward. Keep your arms straight and guide the weights as closely down the front of your balancing leg as possible to protect your back. Maintain a straight/flat back during the entire movement, and keep your shoulders back so they do not roll forward. Once a stretch is felt in the back of your balancing leg, pause, then rotate around the hip back up to your starting position while keeping most of your body weight in your heel. Keep your hips as level as possible throughout the movement. Repeat on the same side for the specified number of repetitions, then switch to the other leg.

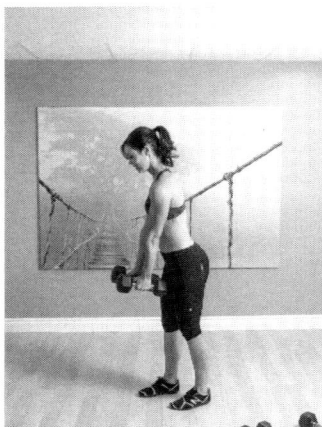

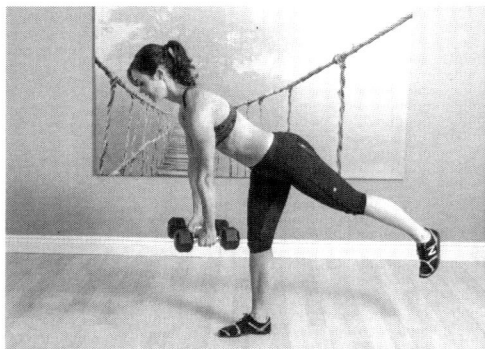

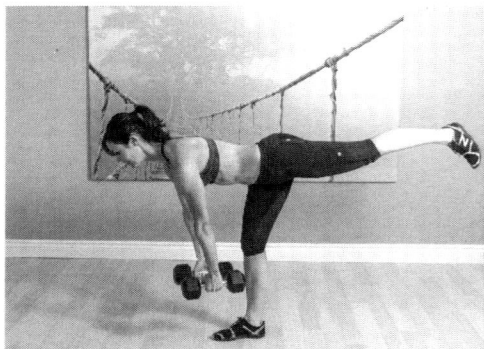

SKIER OVER YOGA MAT

Appears in: Sweaty Intervals #4
Targeted Muscles: Front & back of legs; Buttocks; Calves; Your heart!

Stand on one side of a yoga mat (be sure the yoga mat is not going to slide on the floor and be a slipping risk). If you don't have a yoga mat, put a couple pieces of tape on the floor about two feet apart. From the side of your mat (or tape), jump with both feet to the other side, landing on both feet simultaneously. Repeat this jumping movement back and forth as quickly as you can for the specified amount of time.

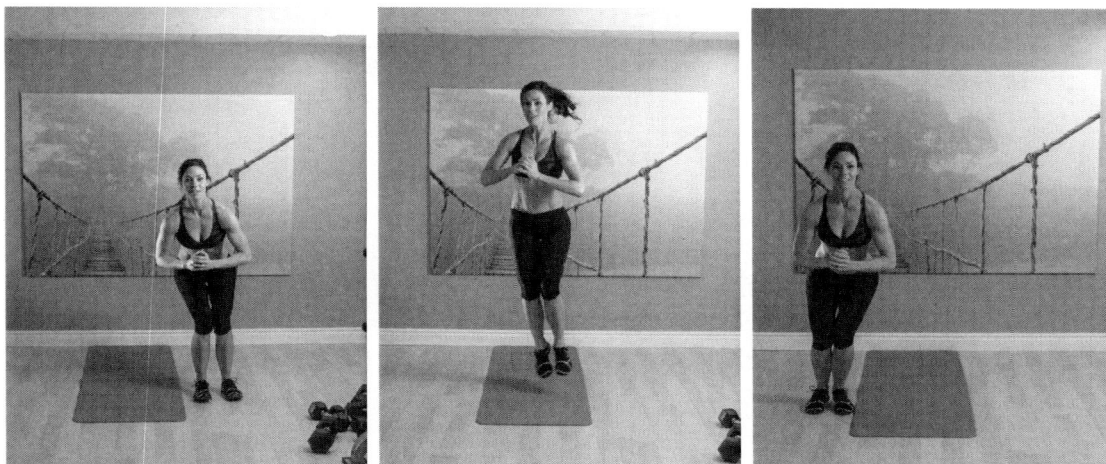

SKIPPING

Appears in: Super Pump #3
Targeted Muscles: Shoulders; Abdominals; Legs; Calves; Your heart!

Skip or jump in place with both feet at the same time. This can be performed with a skipping/jump rope, or you can mimic the rope turning motion with your hands (to keep the arms engaged) if you do not have a rope or enough room to use a rope. Repeat as quickly as you can for the specified amount of time.

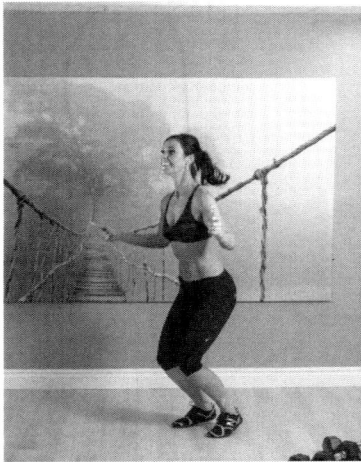

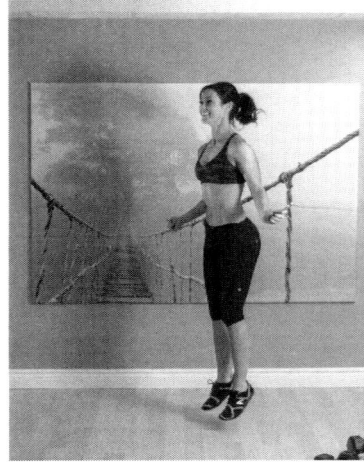

SPIDER JUMP PUSHUPS (PHOTOS ON NEXT PAGE)

Appears in: Killer #8
Targeted Muscles: Shoulders; Upper back; Abdominals; Chest; Side of torso

In a plank off your toes, place your hands just slightly wider than shoulder-width apart. With a tight core (tilt your tailbone toward the floor), jump your right foot up to the outside of your right hand, then jump the right foot back to centre. Repeat the jump sequence with the left foot. From here, complete one pushup. Complete the series (one jump up to your right hand, back, one jump up to your left hand, back, then pushup) for the specified number of repetitions.

SPIDER JUMP PUSHUPS (CONTINUED)

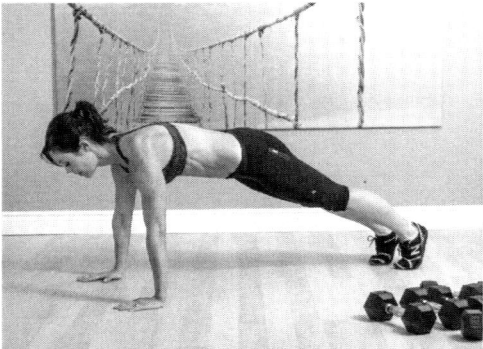

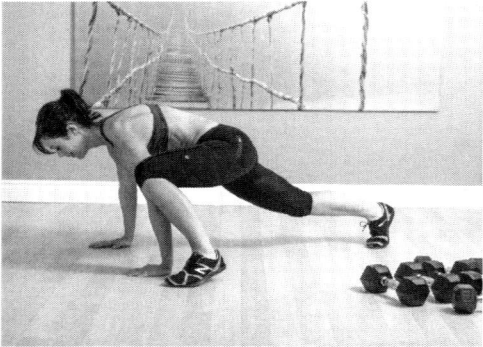

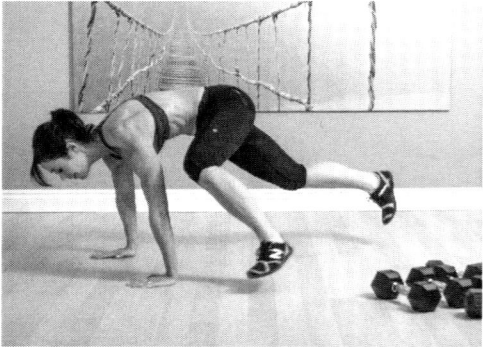

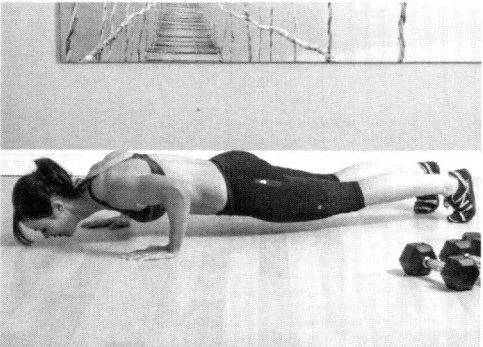

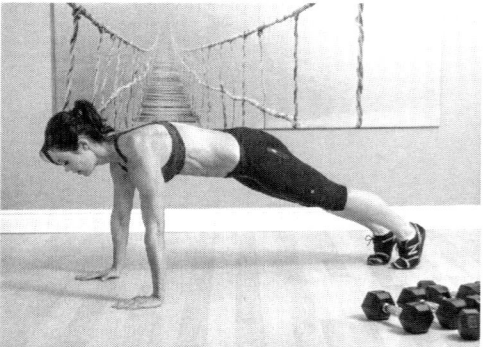

SQUATS (CAN BE COMPLETED WITH OR WITHOUT WEIGHT)

Appears in: Killer #1; Super Pump #1
Targeted Muscles: Front & back of legs; Buttocks

Stand with your feet shoulder-width apart (the inside of your foot should be in line with the outside of your shoulder). Bend at your hips and knees to lower into a squat position (as if you're about to sit in a chair) until your thighs are just past parallel to the floor. If you have knee problems, do not go past parallel. Keep your knees over top of your ankles (you should be able to see your toes throughout the entire movement). Maintain good posture by keeping your chest up as high as you can as you lower into the squat and while you stand back up to complete each repetition.

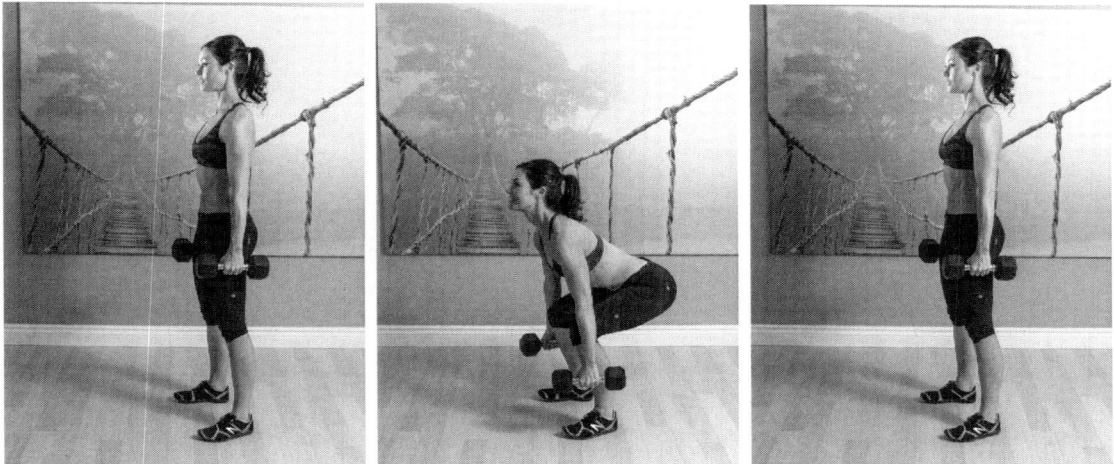

SQUAT DIAGONAL PRESS

Appears in: Killer #5; Super Pump #3
Targeted Muscles: Front & back of legs; Buttocks; Shoulders; Abdominals;
Upper back; Front & back of arms

Stand with your feet shoulder-width apart. Hold a single weight with both your hands and bend your hips and knees into a squat position. Keep your knees behind your toes and your chest up. Push through your heels and stand back up. Rotate to one side and press the weight upward at a 45-degree angle while turning the hips and lifting the back heel up off the floor. Return to centre and go immediately back into a squat position. Complete the specified number of repetitions on one side, then switch to the other side.

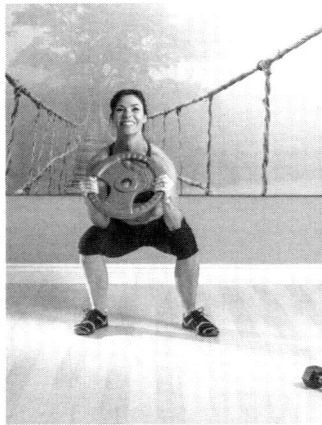

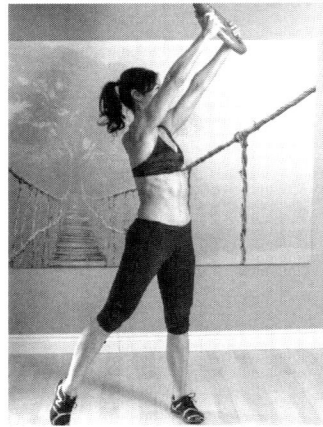

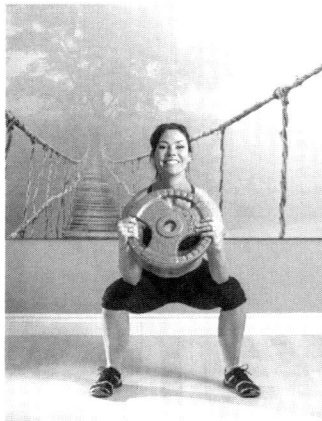

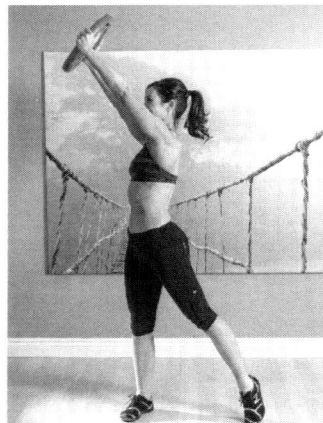

REALITY FITNESS

SQUAT PRESS

Appears in: Killer #3
Targeted Muscles: Front & back of legs; Buttocks; Shoulders; Abdominals

Stand with your feet shoulder-width apart and with a dumbbell in each hand, arms at your sides. Bend at your hips and knees to lower into a squat position until your thighs are just past parallel to the floor. If you have knee problems, do not go past parallel. As you stand back up, bring the weights up to your shoulders, and then press the dumbbells above your head simultaneously. Bring them back down to your sides to squat again.

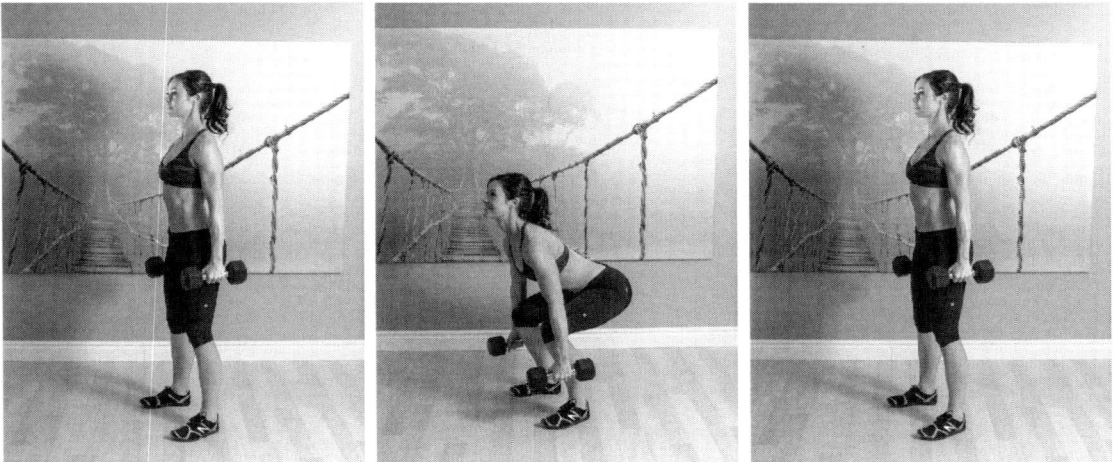

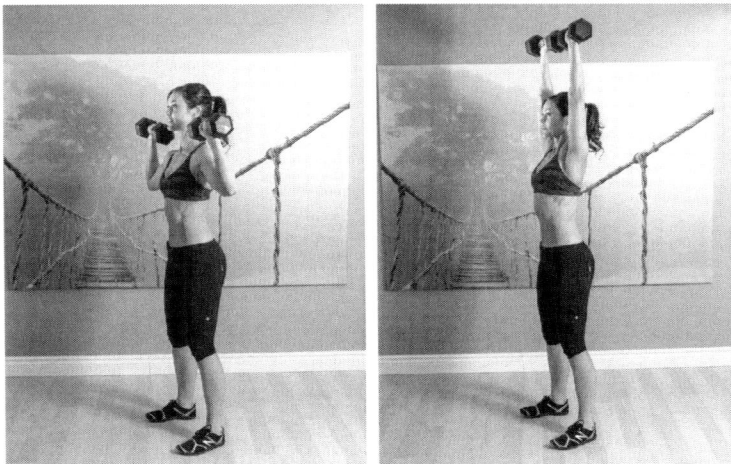

SQUAT WITH V-PRESS

Appears in: Killer #7

Targeted Muscles: Front & back of legs; Buttocks; Shoulders; Abdominals;
Upper back

Stand with your feet shoulder-width apart and with a dumbbell in each hand at shoulder height. Bend your hips and knees to lower into a squat position until your thighs are just past parallel to the floor. If you have knee problems, do not go past parallel. As you stand back up, press the dumbbells above your head into a V position, and then bring them back down to your shoulders to repeat the squat again.

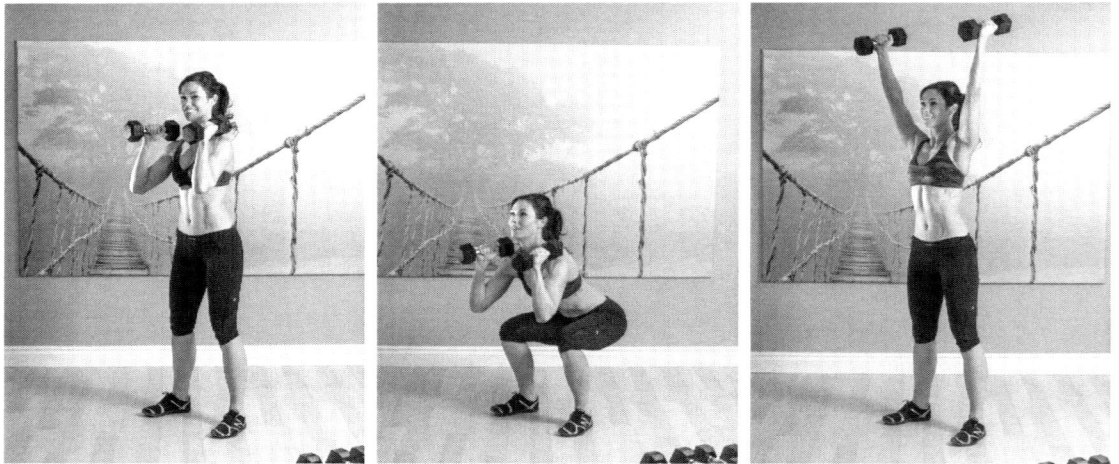

STATIC LUNGE W/ WEIGHTED ARM ROTATION

Appears in: Killer #3
Targeted Muscles: Front, back & inner legs; Buttocks; Calves; Shoulders;
Side of torso; Upper back

Take one large step forward so that when you bend your knees they form two 90-degree angles. Holding a single dumbbell with both hands, extend your arms out in front of you, parallel to the floor. Slowly rotate at the waist over your front knee, keeping both arms extended outwards and your shoulders down (avoid shrugging). Note that your feet do not move during this exercise (which is why it is called "Static"). Rotate back to centre and repeat in the same direction for the specified number of repetitions. Repeat on the other side for the same number of reps.

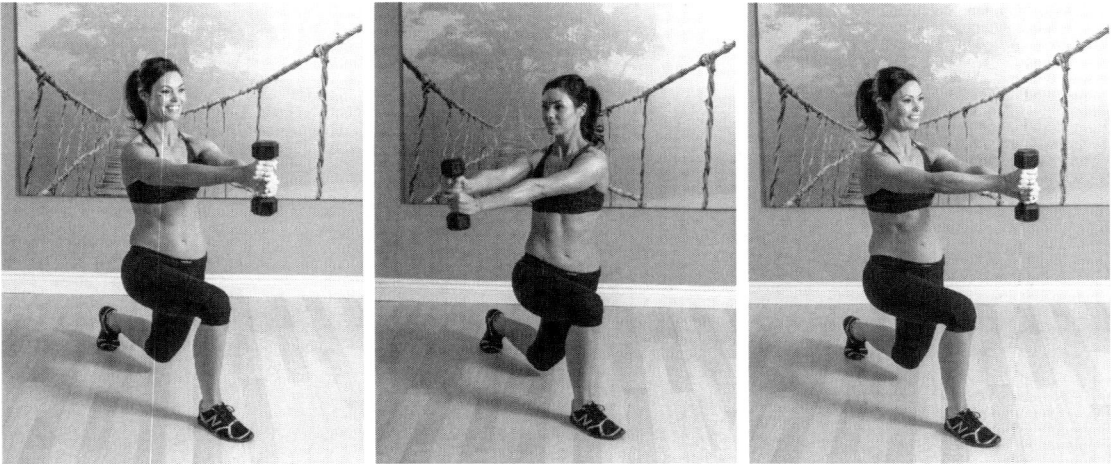

STATIONARY LUNGE WITH PULSES

Appears in: Killer #2
Targeted Muscles: Front & back of legs; Buttocks

Take a large step backward and bend both knees to 90 degrees. Your front knee should track over your front ankle, and your back knee should track underneath your hip and be as close to the floor as possible without touching it. Slowly pulse up and down one to two inches, pushing up slightly from your front heel. Keep the motion controlled and slow. Complete for the specified number of pulses.

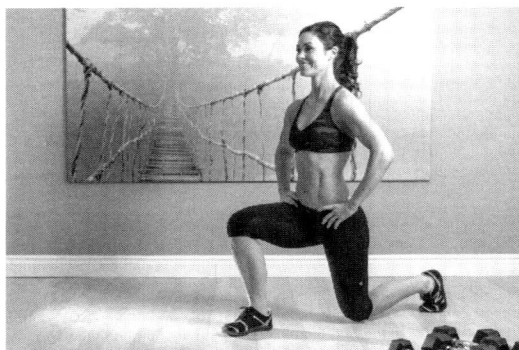

SURRENDERS (PHOTOS ON NEXT PAGE)

Appears in: Killer #3

Targeted Muscles: Front & back of legs; Buttocks; Shoulders; Abdominals;
Upper back

Stand with your feet shoulder-width apart. Holding a weight in each hand (palms facing each other), raise both your arms above your head. Keep your shoulders down away from your ears and maintain straight arms. Keeping your chest up, slowly kneel down onto your knees one leg at a time, leading with your right leg first. Stand back up one leg at a time, again leading with the right leg. When standing up, push through the heel of your foot to engage your buttock muscles and to keep your knee tracking over your ankle, not your toe. Continue this pattern for the specified number of repetitions, and then repeat leading with your left leg.

SURRENDERS (CONTINUED)

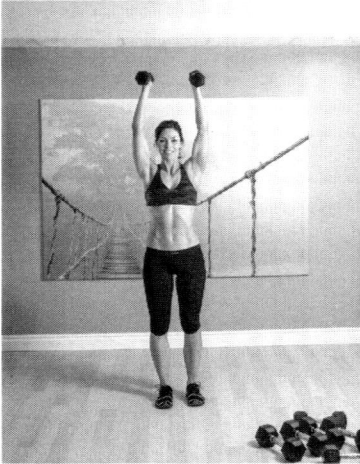

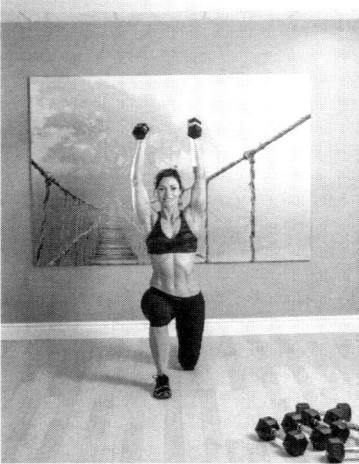

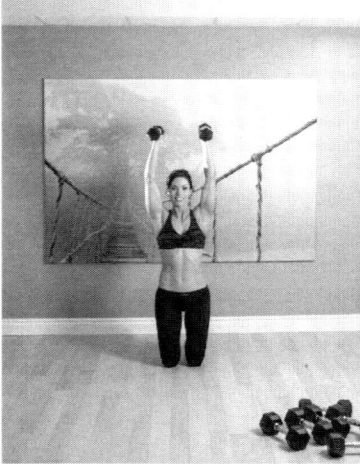

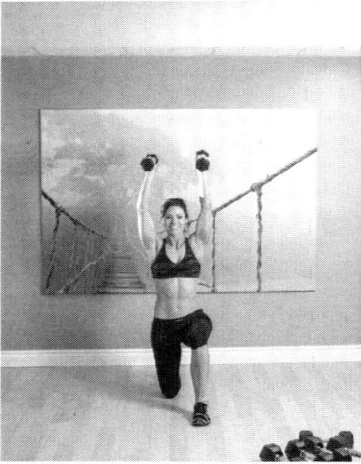

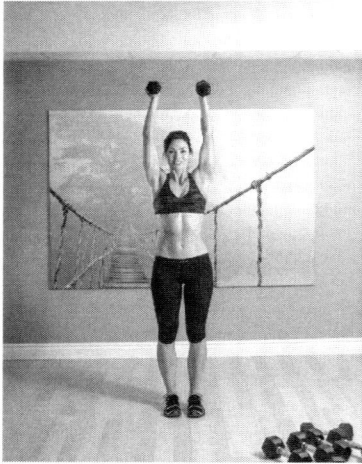

REALITY FITNESS

TOE TOUCHES

Appears in: Killer #2
Targeted Muscles: Front & back of legs; Buttocks; Calves

Stand on one foot with your other leg bent behind you at approximately 90 degrees. Slowly bend your standing leg at the knee and then bend forward at the hip to reach for the floor with both hands while maintaining a flat back. Gently touch the floor, and then slowly stand back up. Complete for the specified number of repetitions, and then repeat on the other side.

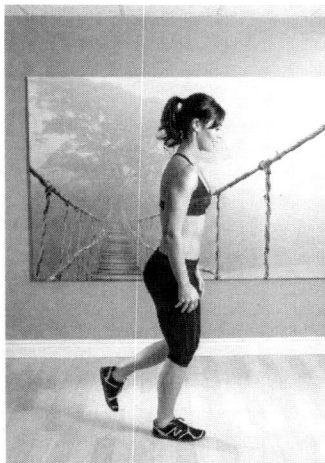

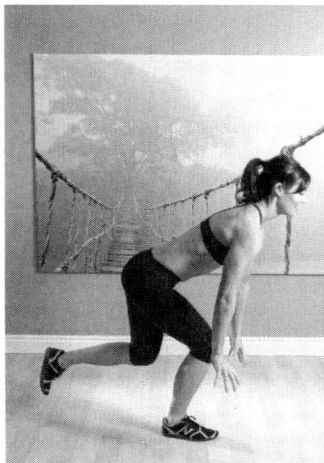

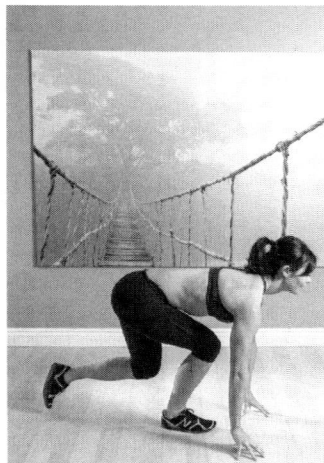

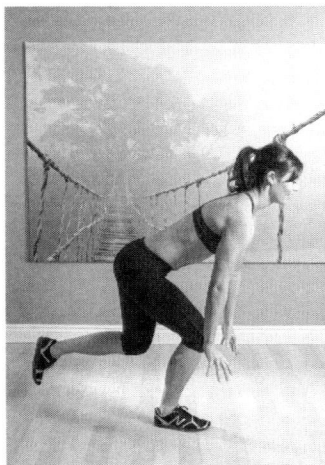

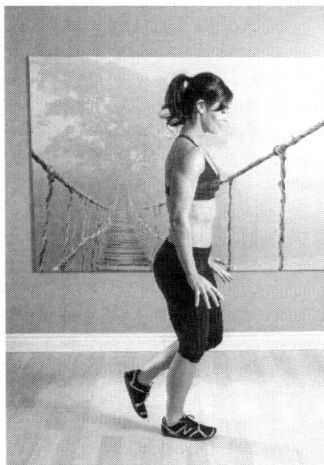

TRANSITION LUNGES

Appears in: Killer #5
Targeted Muscles: Front & back of legs; Buttocks; Calves; Your heart!

Start with both feet together. Take a large step forward into a lunge position, remembering to keep your knee tracking over your ankle. Push off your front heel and transition into a back lunge. Repeat this process—front lunge, into a back lunge, into front lunge, etc.—for the specified amount of time.

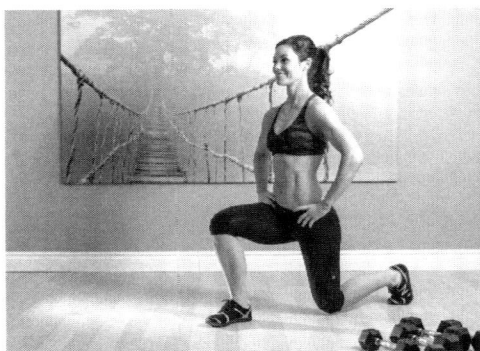

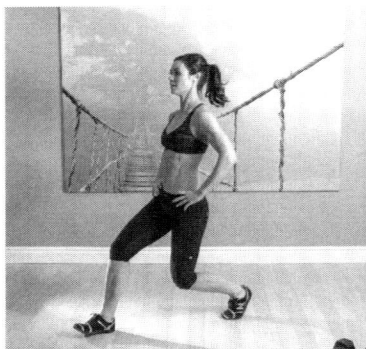

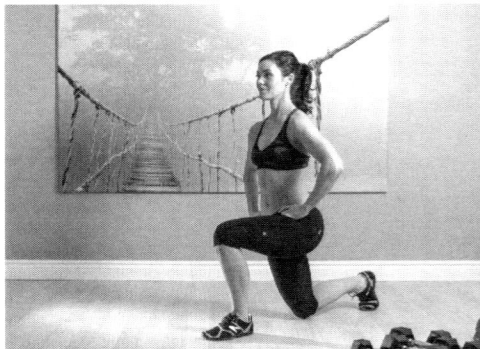

WALKING FRONT LUNGE WITH ROTATION

Appears in: Killer #6
Targeted Muscles: Front, back, & inner legs; Buttocks; Calves; Shoulders;
Upper back; Side of torso

From standing, take one large step forward so that when you bend your knees they form two 90-degree angles. Holding a dumbbell in the centre with both hands, extend your arms out so that they are parallel to the floor. Rotate at the waist over your front knee, keeping your arms extended outwards. Slowly rotate back to centre. Take another step forward and rotate to the other side. As you stand up from each lunge, be sure to push through your front heel to keep your front knee over your front ankle. Continue to perform walking lunges, rotating over each knee as you go, for the specified amount number of repetitions.

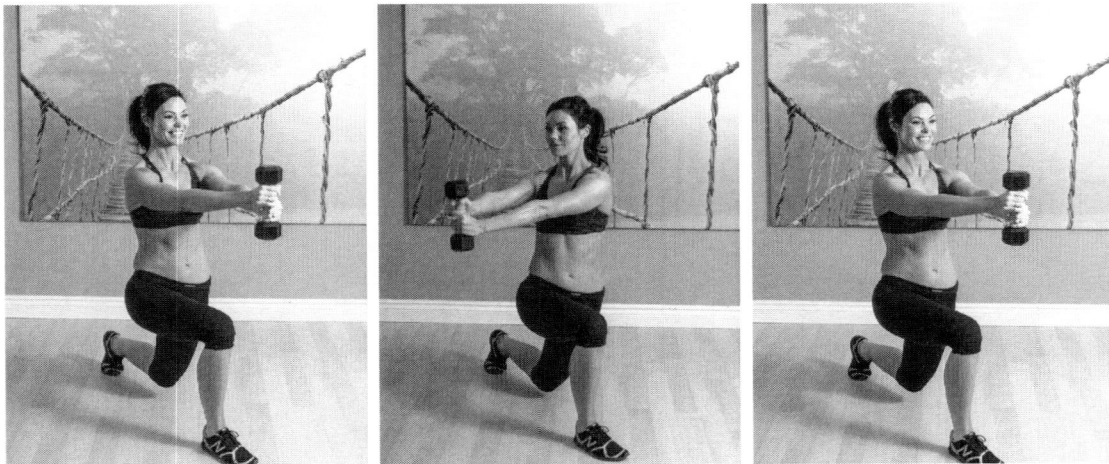

WALKOUTS

Appears in: Killer #2
Targeted Muscles: Shoulders; Abdominals; Chest; Upper back

Start in a standing position. Bend at the waist and place your hands on the floor (if necessary, bend your knees slightly). Once your hands are on the floor, slowly walk one hand out at a time until your back is parallel to the floor (a plank position with your hands located directly under your shoulders). Pause, then walk one hand at a time back toward your feet. Once you reach your feet, stand back up.

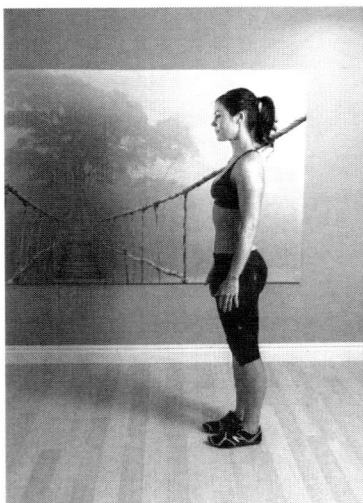

Start and end each rep of this exercise standing up.

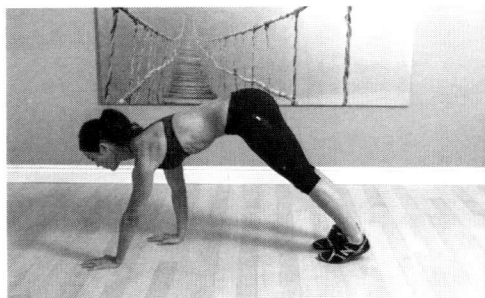

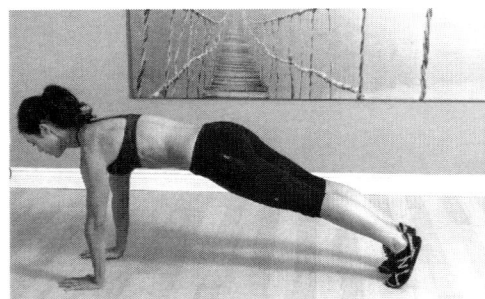

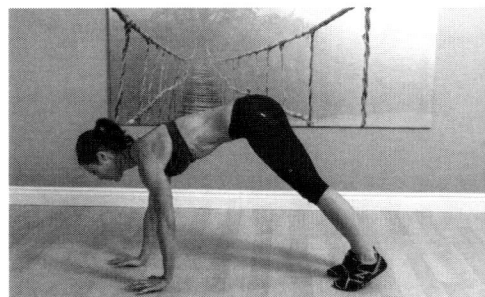

WEIGHTED PUNCHES

Appears in: Sweaty Intervals #1, #2, #3, #4
Targeted Muscles: Shoulders; Upper back; Side of torso; Front & back of arms;
Your heart!

Stand with your feet shoulder-width apart. With two lighter dumbbells in each hand, mimic a punching motion, letting your torso twist as you punch one arm out at a time. Keep a slight bend in your elbows at the end of each punch to avoid over extension. Keep your shoulders down. Repeat as quickly as you can for the specified amount of time.

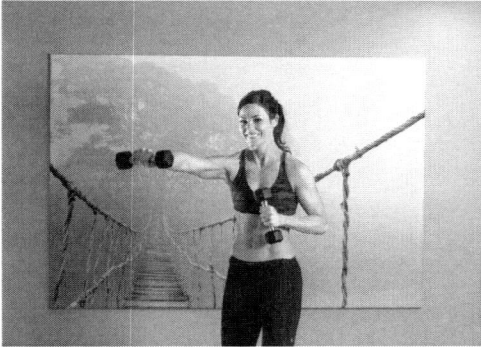

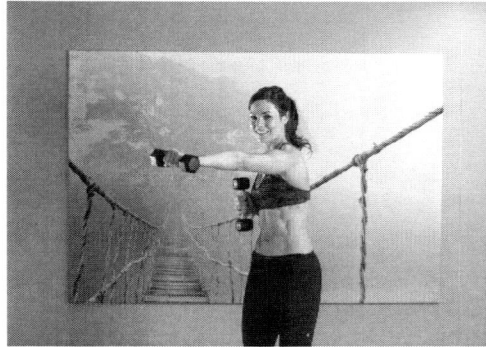

WIDE JUMP SQUATS/LOW JACKS

Appears in: Sweaty Intervals #2, #3, #4
Targeted Muscles: Front, back & inner legs; Buttocks; Calves; Your heart!

Start in a squat position (see Base Squat to review). From the squat, jump up into a standing position with both feet together. From the standing position, jump back into a squat position. Keep your chest up during the entire movement. Repeat as quickly as you can for the specified amount of time.

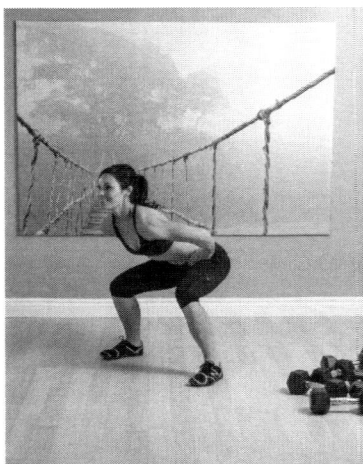

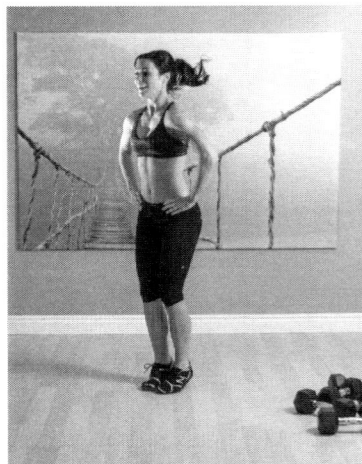

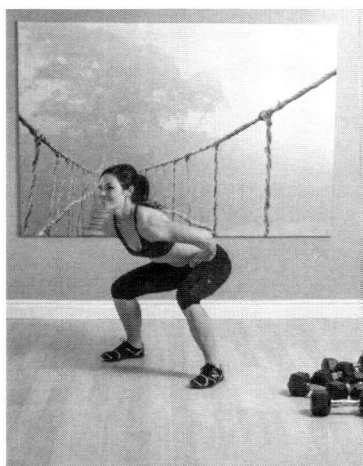

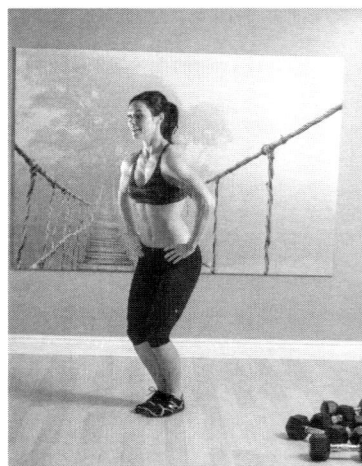

APPENDIX C: FORMS AND CHARTS

PDF downloads of the forms and charts to print or to pull up
on your favourite device are available at:
www.realityfitnessbook.com

REALITY FITNESS NUTRITION AND WORKOUT TRACKER

	Week:								Week:							
	Weight:								Weight:							
Phase	Mon	Tue	Wed	Thu	Fri	Sat	Sun	Mon	Tue	Wed	Thu	Fri	Sat	Sun	80%
N1: 3L Water															
N2: Breakfast															
N3: Eat 3-4 hrs															
N4: Portions															
N5: Veggies															
N6: Protein															
N7: Fat															
N8: Carbs															
N9: Colours															
N10: Natural Food															
10,000 steps															
Workouts															
Celly Countdown		2	1						2	1					

Comments:

	BUILDING	INTENSIFY	ADVANCED	SUSTAINABILITY	
DATE OF ASSESSMENT					
TIME OF DAY					
BODY COMPOSITION					
Weight					
Neck					
Shoulders					
Chest					
Waist					
Hips					
Right Arm					
Right Leg					
CARDIOVASCULAR FITNESS					
1.5 mile run time					
OR					
1.0 mile walk time					
MUSCULAR ENDURANCE					
Squats (# in 1 minute)					
Pushups Off Toes (max #)					
OR					
Pushups Off Knees (max #)					
Plank off Elbows (max time)					
BALANCE					
Right Foot Hops (# in 1 min)					
Left Foot Hops (# in 1 min)					
OR					
Right Foot Standing (max time)					
Left Foot Standing (max time)					
NOTES					

REALITY FITNESS ASSESSMENT TRACKING FORM

REALITY FITNESS PROTEIN | CARB | FAT OPTIONS & PORTIONS

BEST PROTEIN SOURCES

(eat at every snack and meal)

- Beef — 3-4 oz
- Bison — 3-4 oz
- Chicken — 3-4 oz
- Cottage Cheese — ½ cup
- Crab — 3-4 oz
- Eggs — 2
- Egg Whites — 4
- Fish (white fish, tilapia, halibut) — 3-4 oz
- Greek Yogurt (plain) — ½ cup
- Protein Powder (Whey and Casein) — 1 scoop
- Salmon — 3-4 oz
- Scallops — 5 large
- Shrimp — 5 large
- Tofu — ½ cup
- Turkey — 3-4 oz

NEXT BEST PROTEIN SOURCES

- Beans — ½ cup
- Edamame — ½ cup
- Farro — ½ cup
- Hemp Hearts — 2 tbsp
- Lentils — ½ cup
- Nuts — ¼ cup
  (unsalted, unroasted, pistachios, almonds, cashews, macadamia, brazil, pecans, walnuts)
- Nut Butters — 1 tbsp
  (almond, peanut, cashew)
- Seeds — 2 tbsp
  (unsalted, unroasted, sunflower, chia)

BEST GRAIN & OTHER CARBOHYDRATE SOURCES

(eat at breakfast and after workouts)

- Ancient Grains — 1/3 cup uncooked
  (amaranth, barley, farro, millet, quinoa, spelt, teff)
- Apples — 1
- Bananas — 1
- Berries — ½ cup
- Breads — 1 slice
  (pumpernickel, sourdough, whole grain, ezekiel)
- Brown Rice — ½ cup cooked
- Grapefruit — ½
- Oatmeal — ½ cup cooked
- Sweet Vegetables — ¾ cup
  (beets, butternut squash, carrots, corn, parsnips, peas, potatoes, sweet potatoes, tomato sauce, turnips, vegetable juice)
- Tortilla — 1 (6-inch)

BEST FAT SOURCES

(eat at every snack and meal)

- Avocado — 2 tbsp
- Cheese — 1 oz
- Flax (ground) — 1 tbsp
- Nuts — ¼ cup
- Nut Butter — 1 tbsp
- Oils (coconut, grapeseed, olive) — 1 tbsp
- Salad Dressings — 1 tbsp

ACKNOWLEDGMENTS

This book was nearly five years in the making. It would have never happened if it were not for my favourite dad. His trust in my step-by-step nutrition approach and his dedication to the program was the entire inspiration for *Reality Fitness*.

Thank you, Favourite Dad, for opening up, brainstorming, editing along the way, and for allowing me to share your story. Your success has already inspired others to lose weight, get healthy, and change their lives. I'm so proud of what you have accomplished.

Thank you to my Favourite Mom, Favourite Brother, friends, and extended family. Words cannot express how grateful I am to have you in my life. Your continuous support of me, Acacia Fitness, and *Reality Fitness* has been so meaningful. I am so grateful for your love and support.

Mike, my amazing husband and best friend, my absence has been great for your golf game, but I know it has taken some patience and understanding to see this project to the end. You've been supportive, invested in the process, and an incredible listening ear. You continue to encourage my crazy dreams and accept me for who I am. Thank you so much for believing in me.

Thank you Erinne Adachi, who was Erinne Sevigny when this all began. We've been through several momentous events together in the past couple of years, professionally and personally. Your work ethic and passion for this project, your inquisitive nature that I love so much, your support and encouragement, your honesty, and your friendship have been appreciated more than you could know. Through this experience I have learned so much about the editing process, the publishing industry, and book design. Thank you for an amazing introduction to this writing world.

Amie Flowerday—thanks to all of the fantastic work you do behind the scenes with Acacia Fitness, I had the extra time to write this book in the first place. In addition to all of your support behind the scenes, you are an incredible teammate, coach, and friend. Nobody pushes me out of my comfort zone more than you, and I thank you everyday for it.

Thank you to all the guys that participated in the online pilot projects for *Reality Fitness*. Due to confidentiality I will keep your names to myself, but you know who you are. I am so happy for your newfound health and fitness, and am humbled that you trusted me to take you through this process. Thank you for your belief and commitment in the program. Your suggestions, comments, and positive feedback were invaluable and have shaped the online nutrition-coaching program that aligns with the book.

To all of my clients, I am so grateful to have the opportunity to work with you. Every day I get to wake up and do what I love and spend it with incredible people I enjoy so much. To be on the sidelines watching you push everyday to get stronger and healthier so you can continue to live your lives filled with new experiences and adventure is inspiring and a true joy to be a part of. Thank you for all of your support through the years. Your interest, suggestions, and positivity around this book have meant so much.

Thank you Claudine Lavoie for your incredible fitness photography. You are so good at what you do, and you make an intimidating situation comfortable with your professionalism and genuine kindness. I look forward to working together again soon!

Sheena Ohnysty, thank you for applying my makeup and doing my hair for the book's photo-shoot. You are such a talent! Your positivity and support that morning really helped me be at ease for the photo-shoot and was perhaps more meaningful to me than you might have known.

Nathan Smith, thank you for creating the book cover. Your creativity and excitement about the project were awesome. I love what you came up with!

Megan Evans, thank you for your attention to detail on the manuscript proofread. Your feedback and notes were of great value and even had me laughing at times with your funny commentary.

Paul Adachi, thank you for accepting the "hand model" role for the food portion photos in the book. I think you have a shot at another career, if you want it! I also want to thank you for all of your great insights and feedback along the way with regards to the book.

Thank you Jaouad Takhchi for driving me to a place of tranquility in the Atlas Mountains to write the last few chapters of the book. I'll never forget your kindness and hospitality. I promise to hand deliver a copy of *Reality Fitness* to you soon.

Finally, thank you Joel Harper for taking the time to discuss the publishing process with a Canadian girl that had no idea what she was doing. Your expertise in the fitness industry and your guidance on publishing were appreciated more than you could know.

ABOUT ANGELA DEJONG

Angela deJong, a certified personal trainer and owner of Acacia Fitness, graduated from the University of Alberta with a degree in kinesiology. She has been training clients since 2001 and has worked nationally and internationally with hundreds of people ranging from armchair sportsmen to high performance athletes. Many of those armchair sportsmen have even become high performance athletes in this time.

While most clients do not aspire to reach high performance level, they do desire to be healthier, fitter, and happier. This is where Ang comes in. She gradually pushes her clients through nutrition coaching and exercise progression, week after week, to make little changes that add up to big results. She has helped clients lose enough weight to be given permission from their physicians to stop taking their diabetes and high blood pressure medications. She has helped clients bounce back after knee, abdominal, back, and shoulder surgeries. She's witnessed how movement can change the life of someone suffering with arthritis or even depression. Angela has provided her clients the confidence to get out and date again, the health to start a family, the mobility to run pain free, the strength to carry their golf clubs 18 holes, the cardiovascular fitness to hike mountains and run marathons, the courage to change careers, and the motivation to continue to do this for the rest of their lives.

"Fitness is about freedom. A fit body and mind give you the confidence to try just about anything. My clients are doing things they only dreamed they would be doing. It's the best part of my job." - Angela

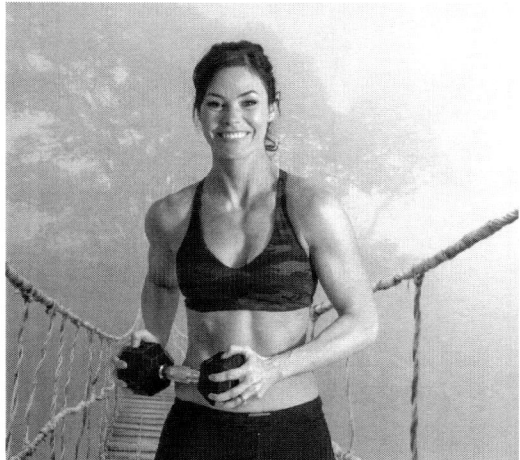

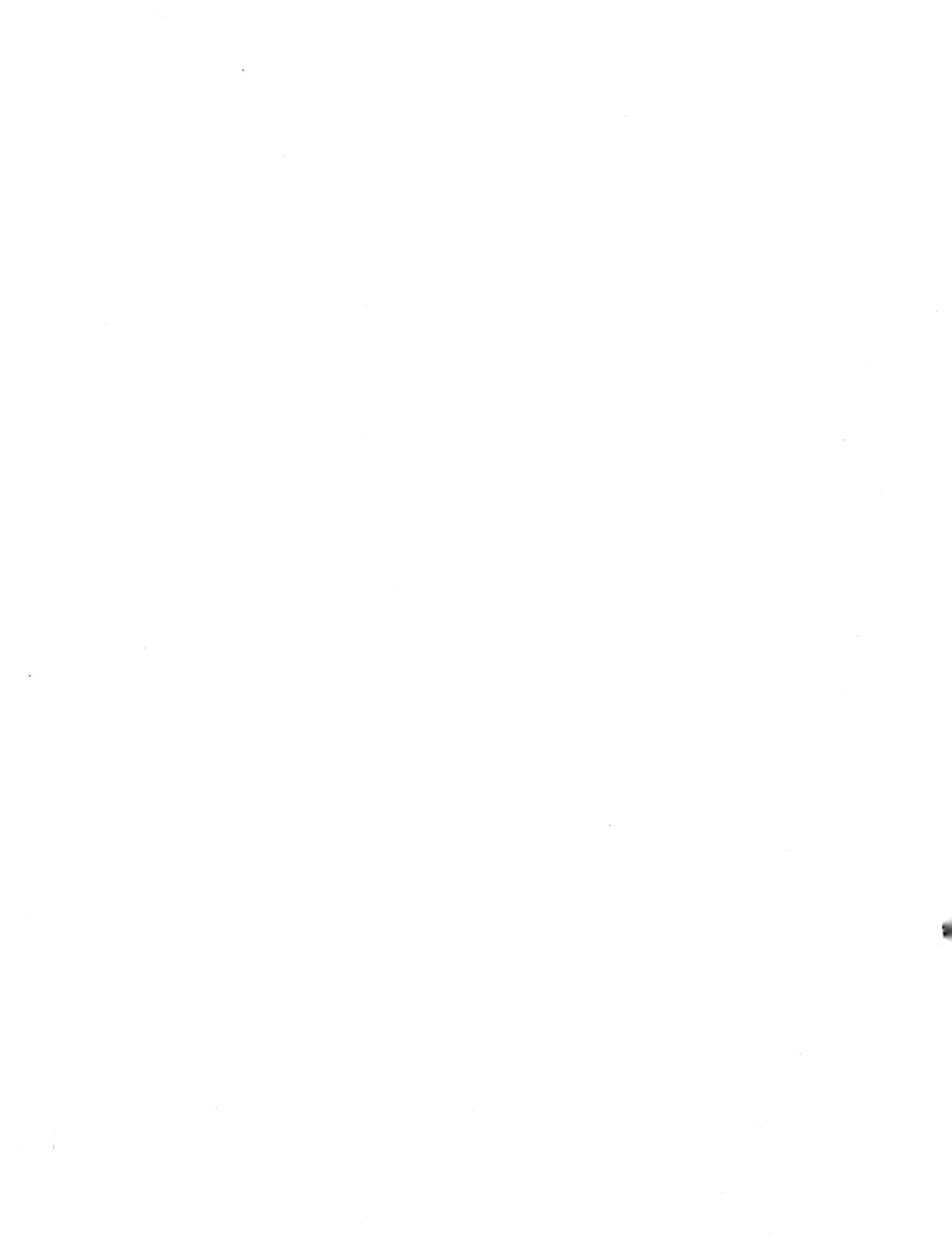